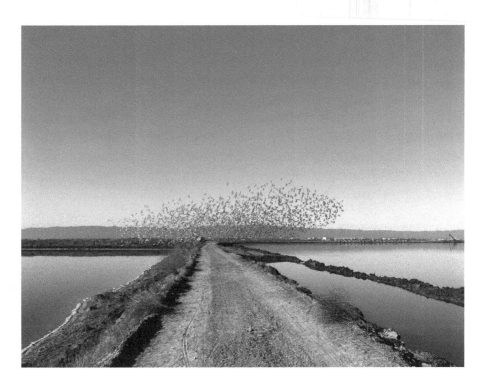

Life Lessons on the Run:
MAKING EVERY STEP COUNT

FIRST EDITION

Cover design by : Amy Sirota

ISBN: 978-0-578-91221-9

Library of Congress Control Number: 2021910156

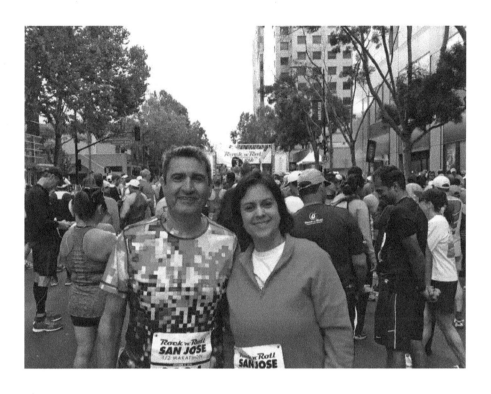

For my biggest fan, my wife

Dear 🌑😊😊 Doc,

peace on trails

Esmail
Nov. 2021

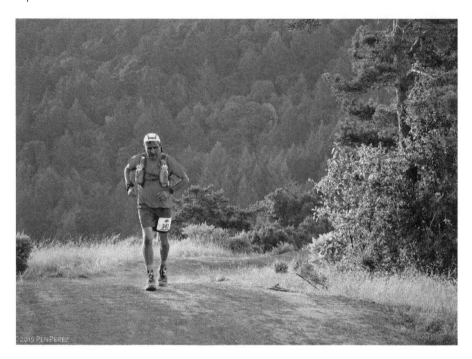

Author's Note

This is a work of nonfiction. The events and experiences described herein are true and have been rendered as I have remembered them, to the best of my knowledge. Some names and identifying details have been changed to protect the privacy of the various people involved.

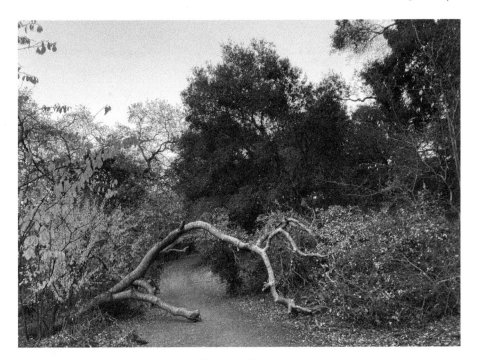

Acknowledgment

I would like to express my gratitude to all the runners who show up for the event, put one foot in front of the other, and then one more step on the roads and trails. Their respect for other beings and nature is an inspiration. Thanks to the San Jose Fit runners for their feedback on the next book they wanted to read, and the support of the 50 States Marathon Club on my goal of completing a marathon in every state and DC. I am grateful to my Tai Chi instructor, Senior Grand Master Ron Lew who provided guidance on incorporating the practice into my runs and healed me from many running injuries.

This book has been in the works for more than a decade. I would like to express special thanks to Priyanka Samant who read my initial stories and provided valuable feedback; to my editor, Jane (Juanita) Usher who patiently read each line of this book and mentored me through the process, to Yeganeh Modirzadeh for the first reading, to Chie Kawahara for her support, and my family for being at the finish line of many races in different seasons.

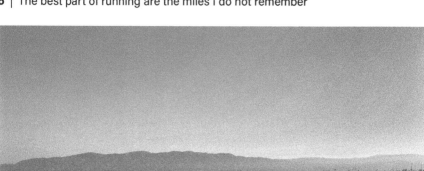

The best part of running are the miles I do not remember

I studied leadership and human behavior as part of my doctorate work and employ those theoretical principals in my professional life. For 26 years, I taught courses on these subjects at various graduate schools of business. In addition, I have led my own businesses for over 30 years. Running, as a hobby, has provided me with an opportunity to travel and meet some of the most interesting people all over the globe. It has also allowed me to utilize what I have studied, taught, and practiced during these experiences.

In my stories, I reflect on how I began racing in 2001 and, so far, have completed over 50 half marathons and over 300 Marathons and ultras. I finished my 50 Sates and DC marathons on June 1, 2014 in Deadwood, South Dakota and completed my goal of racing on all the continents in Morocco on January 25, 2015. The most challenging races so far have been in Death Valley and Antarctica. Although I have traveled to many places to race, my favorite marathon course remains the Napa Valley Marathon in California, where I ran my first marathon.

The stories in this collection are reflections of my encounters and I am grateful for the lessons learned. I have learned that most distance runners do not necessarily have the healthiest hearts. I have witnessed many fatalities during races linked to heart issues which may not have been diagnosed as a pre-existing condition. Race directors of major races have begun highlighting these issues by having runners sign releases of liability specific to heart conditions. My own experience with heart disease, and how my doctors missed all the signs of a 95% blockage on my right main artery, is detailed in my story the "Heart of Hearts."

Running and racing on the trails have taught me how to have a greater deal of respect for nature. I have raced in extreme conditions and learned how to better listen to my body. My encounters with wildlife, from mountain lions on the trails near our home in Los Gatos, California, to an encounter with moose and being chased by bears in Alaska while avoiding variety of snakes in different trail regions, have been a constant reminder that I am a guest in their territory.

I enjoy trail running and, currently, am mostly interested in ultra-racing. I practice meditative running, Zen walks, yoga and core strength. I also practice and teach Tai-Chi and Qigong. Incorporating their principals has taught me how to transform my running into "mediation in motion" by silencing my mind, being present and connecting with the energy of the earth. Mastery of the game is my motivation.

In the early years of racing, I tried answering the question of why I run to my friends and family. Countless hours of training and about a100 races later, I realized that birds do not think of flying and fish do not see the water they swim in. Running is as natural to me as breathing, but it has also been a humbling experience. It has taught me to show up for the events in my life, put one foot in front of the other, make mistakes, embrace the situation and be grateful for the lessons learned. The hardest part of racing these days is getting to the start line. The best parts are the miles I do not remember.

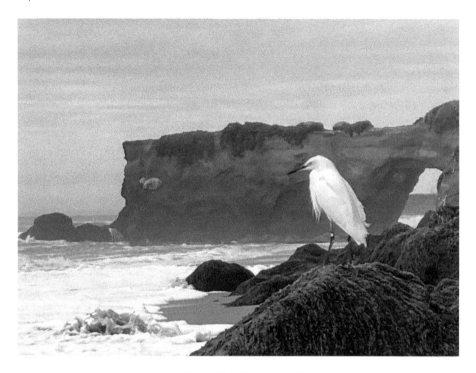

How It All Started

Is it about the journey and not the destination? With no training or preparation, I began running again in the spring of 2001 during the Wharf to-Wharf race in Santa Cruz, California. I had just dropped off a few friends at the start of the race when they asked me to join them on the six-mile run from the Boardwalk in Santa Cruz to the shores of Capitola. My main concern was how we would get back to the car afterward. They said we would worry about it when we finished the race.

It had been over 22 years since I had run cross-country in college. After spending many hours in the library at school, I would rush to my apartment to change and go for a run around the neighborhood before dark. Those easy runs helped to clear my mind and gave me a better focus on my studies. In those days, I never had the urge to participate in any races.

After college in the mid 1980s, I stopped running but continued to stay active by playing racquetball regularly. In the 1990s I also joined a judo club. The many injuries I sustained from years of judo competitions eventually convinced me to seek other sports. My discovery of yoga and meditation healed some of the injuries; however, concussions, broken ribs and a collapsed lung from judo continue to haunt me to this day.

In the late 1990s, I discovered Tai Chi to be a great challenge and that was enough motivation to master this form of martial art. I was fortunate to be trained by Senior Grand Master Ron Lew. He witnessed my frustration and slow progress for a couple of years before calling me aside and informing me that he decided to accept me as a student. Once accepted as a student, the Senior Grand Master also taught me Qigong, Stick Fighting techniques, and Katana Sword.

It was during this time that I ran the Wharf-to-Wharf. Standing in the energy of the large crowd at the start of the race in spring of 2001, I figured why not? I had shown up to the event as a guest, but I decided to accept the challenge and give it a try. I remember that it was a beautiful day to run, the morning dawned clear and cool. The spectators were incredibly enthusiastic. I found the first few miles difficult to run since there were at least 12,000 people jostling one another in the narrow residential streets of Santa Cruz and Capitola. Since I had joined spontaneously, all I had on were jeans, a short sleeve dress shirt and regular shoes. I had no running gear, did not have a bib and ran the race unofficially. I ran hard and was pretty sore when I completed the race. My feet hurt from running in dress shoes. A couple of friends who had completed the race ahead of me cheered me through the finish line. I found it exciting to watch for more friends while they finished their race and we celebrated together. One of my friends gave me her finisher's T-shirt as a souvenir; I must still have it somewhere in my pile of race shirts. Our conversation over a slice of pizza at the finish revolved around how to get the car we had left near the start. I must have still been buoyed up by my "runner's high" because I volunteered to run the course backward to get the car. As I ran, I encouraged the last runners going toward the finish line. By the time I arrived at the beginning of the race, they were removing the cones marking the course and opening the roads to traffic.

Reflecting on this exhilarating experience a few weeks later, I figured that I should be able to run a half marathon with some training and consider running longer distance races in the future. The stress of my work life was at its peak and running helped me to slow down and relax. I started training a few weeks later, ran the Silicon Valley Half Marathon in San Jose, California in the fall of 2001. I started training for a full marathon a couple of weeks later. In March of 2002, with my family waiting for me at the finish line, I ran the Napa Valley marathon in California. I was officially hooked on distance running.

My Senior Grand Master played a pivotal role in my training for races. He taught me how to incorporate the principals of my martial arts practice into my running. After each class we would dissect my previous race with respect to my learnings of Qi and set new strategies for the upcoming races. At the same time, the Senior Grand Master cured my running-related injures through Qigong Energy Healing techniques. I learned how to bring the mindfulness practice into my running, thereby running became meditation in motion. These practices gave me the tools to race marathons and/or ultras every weekend. A decade after I was accepted as a student, I was honored to earn my Tai Chi teacher certification. I have continued with the practice of Qigong and Tai Chi as an instructor.

This is how I got back into running and racing 22 years after completing college. Over the years, I returned to the site of my first marathon in Napa to run my 100th, 150th, and 250th marathons and ultras with old and new running friends. Running the same course always brings back memories of that first 26.2-mile race from Calistoga to Napa in California. I credit the Wharf to-Wharf with restarting my running regimen and honor its place in my life. Through the years, I have run the race many times with my family. We have dragged our sons half asleep to the start of the race from a very young age, and this race remains one of their favorite annual events.

First Race
Wharf to Wharf
April 2001

Wharf to Wharf Race - is a 6-mile footrace from the Santa Cruz Wharf to the Capitola Wharf.
https://raceroster.com/events/2019/22431/wharf-to-wharf-race-2019#:~:text=The%20
Wharf%20to%20Wharf%20Race,running%20of%20the%20iconic%20event

Tai Chi - is an internal Chinese martial art practiced for both its defense training and its health benefits. But it has been part of Chinese martial arts culture since the 16th Century.
https://www.bbc.com/news/world-asia-china-39853374#:~:text=Tai%20Chi%20is%20an%20
internal,culture%20since%20the%2016th%20Century

Qigong - is an ancient Chinese healing art involving meditation, controlled breathing, and movement exercises
https://www.merriam-webster.com/dictionary/qigong

Stick Fighting - is a variety of martial arts which use simple long slender, blunt, hand-held, generally wooden «sticks» for fighting; such as a staff, cane, walking stick, baton, or similar weapons.
https://en.wikipedia.org/wiki/Stick-fighting

Katana - A long, curved single-edged sword traditionally used by Japanese samurai.
https://www.dictionary.com/browse/katana

Runner's high - A feeling of euphoria that is experienced by some individuals engaged in strenuous running and that is held to be associated with a release of endorphins by the brain
https://www.merriam-webster.com/dictionary/runner%27s%20high

Qi - Vital energy that is held to animate the body internally and is of central importance in some Eastern systems of medical treatment (such as acupuncture) and of exercise or self-defense (such as tai chi).
https://www.merriam-webster.com/dictionary/qi

Qigong Healing Technique - Chinese medicine holds that sickness, pain, and other health problems are caused when Qi energy is blocked. Qigong practice removes blocks and increases the flow of energy through your body. When energy flows freely, Qi energy heals and restores the body.
https://www.learningstrategies.com/Qigong/2Level2.asp

Mindfulness - means maintaining a moment-by-moment awareness of our thoughts, feelings, bodily sensations, and surrounding environment, through a gentle, nurturing lens. Mindfulness also involves acceptance, meaning that we pay attention to our thoughts and feelings without judging them—without believing, for instance, that there's a "right" or "wrong" way to think or feel in a given moment. When we practice mindfulness, our thoughts tune into what we're sensing in the present moment rather than rehashing the past or imagining the future.
https://greatergood.berkeley.edu/topic/mindfulness/definition

Ultramarathon - An ultramarathon, also called ultra-distance or ultra-running, is any footrace longer than the traditional marathon length of 42.195 kilometers (26 mi 385 yd).
https://en.wikipedia.org/wiki/Ultramarathon

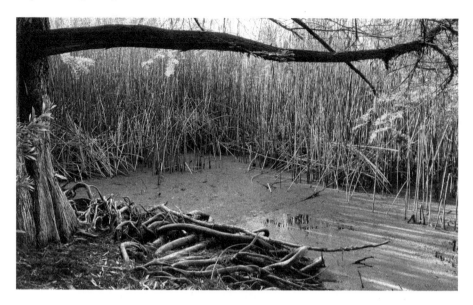

Believing in Myself

Salt Lake City, Utah was cold and crisp in April of 2008. I had hurried from work on a Friday afternoon to get to San Francisco International Airport for my flight there. I was participating in a marathon and needed to make it to the Salt Palace Convention Center for the race expo before it closed. The plane ride gave me the chance to leave work behind in Santa Clara, California and focus on the 26.2-mile race. As soon as I was off the plane, I ran toward a waiting cab and made it to the race expo in time to pick up my race packet and buy souvenirs for my wife and sons. I usually remember the person staffing the booth who hands me my race packet. This time it was a nice older lady. I asked her about the weather for the next day, but she was not sure about the forecast. When I inquired about the location of the start line, she thought maybe it was at the University of Utah, but she did not know. In this case, I remembered her because she was not very helpful, something I found amusing considering the fact she was staffing the race table. To make up for her lack of knowledge, she did think to remind me to read the race schedule for the details before the race.

Admittedly, I had waited until the last minute to find a place to stay and discovered the race-sponsored hotel was sold out, along with all the neighboring hotels in the downtown area. I had managed to book a room at the Guest House of the University of Utah. Imagine my surprise when I read the race schedule and found out that the race began at the University. I could not have been more perfectly placed for the start of the race. This time my procrastination had worked to my advantage.

After I left the race expo I thought about walking to the Guest House with the heavy bag strapped to my shoulder. I was glad that I did not since the Guest House sat on top of a hill. After spending a few minutes looking for a cab, I gave up and walked to a nearby bus stop. With one heavy bag strapped to my shoulder, I listened to detailed instructions from the bus driver on how I did not need his bus; rather I had to catch the trolley that would let me off just two blocks away from the university. I thanked him and told him my hope would be to remember his instructions.

It had been a long time since I had used public transportation and buying a ticket for the trolley became a task. The first self-serve machine would not take my money and, as the line started building behind me, I became flustered and stepped aside. Seeing my dilemma, a nice student walked me to another machine and showed me how to buy a ticket. By then my trolley had come and gone. I did not mind since I was in no hurry to get to the Guest House.

While I waited on the platform across from the House of Kabob and stared down the rails, I began to reminisce about my first train ride thirty years ago from Los Angeles to Oakland, California. Trains were the most popular mode of transportation in Iran, where I am from. That California train ride represented the final leg of my long journey from Tehran, Iran to UC Berkeley.

In 1978, I was an undergraduate student at the Institute of Informatics and Statistics in Tehran. However, at that time Tehran was in a violently escalating situation. With the gradual increase of tension, we were conditioned not to realize the magnitude of the violence around us. I had gotten frustrated with the daily demonstrations against the Shah of Iran that interrupted my classes at the university. That was a big motivation for me to leave home and study abroad. I decided it would be best to continue my education in the United States, the place introduced by Hollywood as the land of milk and honey. Our classes at the university in Tehran were held in English, so I had academic knowledge of the language and figured that would be beneficial at an American university. Getting acceptance letters from well-known universities in the U.S. was the easy part; getting a passport and Visa to the U.S. turned out to be a monumental task that required patience and persistence.

Finally, at age 19, with nothing but a tote bag in my hand, I made it to New York on a windy evening in September of 1978. I had to stay overnight before catching a flight to Los Angeles the following day. I flagged down a taxi outside of JFK Airport and, when he asked me where I needed to go, all I could think of was Harlem. I had no hotel reservations and no idea what Harlem was like in the late 1970's. I ignored the strange look of the taxi driver when I asked him, in my broken English, to please drop me off at a cheap hotel in Harlem. As the saying goes, be careful what you ask for, you may just get it. Trying to understand the thick accent of the clerk at the run-down hotel in Harlem was a challenge, but I welcomed a bed after a long flight crammed into economy class. I crashed only to wake up to popping sounds, like firecrackers, in the street below. These were the familiar sounds of bullets flying around my neighborhood in Tehran in the months before I left for the U.S. Instinctively, I hit the floor and pulled the blanket from the bed to cover myself. I survived the night and happily went to the airport for my flight to Los Angles in the morning.

My final destination was Holy Names College in Oakland, California. I stayed in a dorm at the college and completed many English proficiency classes before attending UC Berkeley. For some reason I had not booked a connecting flight to Oakland from Los Angeles. When I found out the last-minute ticket prices at the airport, I thought it would be best to take the train. I figured this would give me a chance to see the coast from a train window. Somehow, I made it to the Amtrak station and got myself a ticket. Soon the sights of California and the rhythmic sounds of the train mesmerized me; but the cracks of gunfire from Harlem were still ringing in my ears while I sat in the dining car looking at the lunch menu. I remember the lunch included a small salad and the waiter gave me a choice of salad dressings, the names of which I had never heard before. In Iran, we made our own dressings at home and restaurants where I ate did not offer any choices. I asked the waiter to make the choice for me and that was my introduction to the choices of salad dressing, and many more choices to follow. I began to realize that not knowing anyone in the U.S. may not work to my advantage and I knew that my learning curve was going to be pretty steep. Tough experiences that followed, taught me how to believe in myself.

Like everything else I found fresh and fascinating in this land, once I debarked at the Amtrak station in Oakland, I had to stand for a while to take in all the new sights and sounds before asking the ticket desk how to get to my destination. The lady at the counter was kind to understand my limited English and explained very slowly which bus I need to take outside of the station.

I took the bus from the train station and with the help of the bus driver, I learned how a transfer ticket worked. I carefully wrote down the number of the buses I had to transfer to and the names of the stations. The first and second bus drivers were nice to call on me at the transfer stops. The last driver had a thick accent and appeared to be drowned in his thoughts. However, after the second time passing the station by the college, he noticed me and asked why I was riding an empty bus that day. Once he understood my dilemma, he was kind enough to call on me when we got to the stop by the college the third time. With time and practice, my English got better.

In late November of 1978, one of my teachers from San Francisco came into class with wet eyes and told us George Moscone and Harvey Milk were shot that morning at the San Francisco City Hall. For many years, I did not understand what that meant and how that event would impact the country for years to come. I made a few friends along the way and got to explore the hills of Oakland and the neighboring Berkeley on foot. The Iranian student community was sharply divided over the events happening back home and a few of the Berkeley students that I met were calling themselves activists in order to bring change and justice to Iran. The revolution that followed in the spring of 1979 changed the course of history back home and shut the doors for many of students, including me, who once thought we would take our education home and make a change for better in our society.

All of these memories, and those of my family back home, were on my mind as the trolley snaked through downtown Salt Lake City and into the University of Utah. I stepped out at Fort Douglas Station on the University campus and took the short walk toward the Guest House. Going over Victory Bridge, I saw the students setting up a huge American flag on the lawn beneath the bridge by the side of the road in preparation for the marathon. Guest House proved to be nice and clean but, when I asked for restaurants nearby, the nice lady at the front desk told me that the only place within walking distance was the school cafeteria that would close in about 45 minutes. She handed me a small map of the campus with letters in very small fonts that I could hardly read. After dropping my bag in the room, I rushed out the door only to get even more confused by the map in my hand. It was late in the afternoon when I walked outside. Going toward where I thought the cafeteria would be, I heard a live band playing in a gazebo near an open area facing the dorms. When I got closer, I saw there were four students playing their music to no audience. I managed to find three students sitting on a porch and two of them gave me vastly different directions to the cafeteria. I decided to continue walking and asked another student who barely spoke English. He knew enough to say that he had no idea. Finally, I saw a guy kicking back on a bench near what looked like a library. As I got closer, I noticed that he was smoking a joint and traveling in his own universe. I decided to ask him anyways and his response was, "I do not know man." I thought if anyone should know his way to the cafeteria, it would be him. After all, wouldn't the effects of his pot smoking soon call for a trip there to satisfy his "munchies"? After walking around some more, I saw a couple carrying food they had just purchased at the cafeteria. With half an hour left to closing, I made it upstairs to indulge in an "all-you-can-eat" food court. Being hungry, everything looked good. I headed for the nearest sandwich station. When asked what I wanted, I told the server that I was running a marathon the next day and I was at his mercy for a good load of carbohydrates. He asked me the distance of a marathon and I responded 42.2 kilometers. He was delighted that someone else had used the metric measurement because he grew up with it in Poland. While he was making my sweet turkey sandwich (two pieces of bread with mayonnaise, turkey, crushed potato chips and a big squeeze of honey) we talked about the lack of job opportunities in his native country. He told me that, even with a degree, he was forced to come back here to the U.S. to work in a cafeteria. As I walked away, he commented that he could never run a marathon since he was no longer in shape. After eating my tasty sandwich, I could not blame him; if I worked behind that same counter I might also have been out of shape.

Walking out of the cafeteria, I could see downtown Salt Lake City. From my viewpoint at the top of the hill the city gleamed in the sunset. A walkway went down the hill toward the faculty dormitories surrounded by a large expanse of freshly cut lawn. I could picture the students hanging out there on warm days while enjoying the cityscape. It felt serene and peaceful. For a moment I wished my family were there since our young boys would have enjoyed running around on that endless grass.

After a good night's sleep, I made my way to the start, next to the big flag laid in the lawn by the students I saw the day before. The harmonious voices of a large choir singing on top of the bridge above us were the highlight of the start line. Despite periodic dusty winds from the Great Salt Lake, the weather was great. The course changed directions enough that there were good breaks from those pesky gusts. We had a lot of support throughout the whole course; many of the residents of the neighborhoods cheered on the runners, making us feel awesome. I encountered well-stocked aid stations and friendly volunteers. The race officials and the volunteers managed the finish area well; however, the finish line food consisted of an unappetizing hot dog that I found easy to refuse.

The mile-walk back to the Guest House from the finish line helped ease the tension of my sore calf muscles. I took a quick shower, packed, then rushed to get to the airport to catch my flight home. Later, I would find out it is best to get a good night's rest after a race before traveling, especially if flying. I read somewhere that, due to the inflammation of the brain after a marathon, it is best not to fly in order to allow enough time for the swelling to subside. At thirty thousand feet, I was already looking at my calendar and planning the next race. I guess that is what marathon brain inflammation does to me!

Marathon Number 22
Salt Lake City, Utah
April 2008

Informatics - Is the study of computational systems, especially those for data storage and retrieval. (According to ACM Europe and Informatics Europe informatics is synonym for computer science and computing as a profession, in which the central notion is transformation of information.
https://en.wikipedia.org/wiki/Informatics

George Moscone and Harvey Milk - Former Board of Supervisors member Dan White murders Mayor George Moscone and Supervisor Harvey Milk at City Hall in San Francisco, California. White, who stormed into San Francisco's government offices with a .38 revolver, had reportedly been angry about Moscone's decision not to reappoint him to the city board. Firing upon the mayor first, White then reloaded his pistol and turned his gun on his rival Milk, who was one of the nation's first openly gay politicians and a much-admired activist in San Francisco. Future California Senator and then-Supervisor Dianne Feinstein, who was the first to find Milk's body, found herself addressing a stunned crowd at City Hall. "As president of the Board of Supervisors, it's my duty to make this announcement: Both Mayor Moscone and Supervisor Harvey Milk have been shot and killed. The suspect is supervisor Dan White."
https://www.history.com/this-day-in-history/san-francisco-leaders-george-moscone-and-harvey-milk-are-murdered

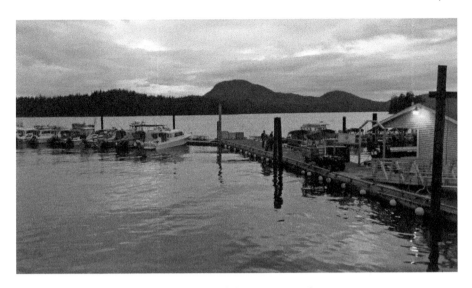

A Moose and her Two Calves

I had run the San Francisco Marathon back in 2004 and remembered there were stretches in Golden Gate Park that were not too appealing. Just the thought of a boring run, starting at mile 13 in Golden Gate Park and lasting to around mile 24 just before AT&T Park, kept me preoccupied. I thought it would be difficult for me to enjoy the serenity of the park anticipating those miles.

Thankfully, a month before the race, I left for a fishing trip in Alaska with a group of friends. It made for a good opportunity to take my mind off of the upcoming race. Little did I know how much of a distraction that trip would be. Our destination was a little fishing town of Gustavus near the Gulf of Alaska, a place I had fished for the last 20 years. The day after we arrived, I went out for a run near our cabin in the woods. It was about four in the morning when I left the cabin and started my run on a dirt road that began right outside of the front door. The night before, we had gone for a hike after dinner and I mapped out my run for the next day. I knew I had to stay in shape for the upcoming San Francisco Marathon. Since there was not much darkness up there in summer, 4:00 a.m. seemed to be a good time to run; it was nice and bright outside with crisp air providing a perfect temperature for running. There were no cars, no bikes and no human beings to be seen for miles. Towering trees surrounded the road but I could still see a good distance into the forest as I looked ahead. The only sounds I could hear were my own footfalls and breathing. Before leaving the cabin, I had grabbed a canister of pepper spray (about the size of a big can of hairspray) to use as a bear repellent. A mile into the run, as I immersed myself in the serenity of the forest, I happened to look to my right and saw a moose with two calves standing about five feet away from the road by a little creek. From their curious looks, I gathered they were wondering who I was and why I was running in their habitat. I had read that moose with calves could be deadly and, if the mother feels the calves are being threatened, their 1,300 pounds of weight can turn a human being into sawdust. I had seen plenty of moose in my prior trips to Alaska and witnessed how fast they could run. My fear set in and a cold sweat followed, but I continued my run since I did not know what else to do at that moment. I did not look back and continued on that scenic road cheered by the surrounding trees. In the back of my mind I had hopes of spotting a car or some sign of human life.

Turning a corner after a few fast miles and seeing more of the lonely dirt road, I remembered that I had sent an email to all my fishing buddies before the trip warning them not to wander outside alone while we were up there. Why did I think I was exempt from this precaution? There I was, alone and holding a can of bear spray, spooking myself with scary thoughts of bears and moose, with no one in sight. This moment of clarity led me to get in touch with my own hypocrisy; for years, the very same thing bothered me when I came across it in others. I should be thankful to that moose for the realization of why hypocrisy had bothered me so much in the past. It presented itself as a kind of entitlement. Another fear owned and lesson to remember from a near-fatal encounter.

Finally, I decided to turn around and head back toward the cabin, knowing the exact spot where I had seen the moose with her calves. As I got closer, I decided not to look for her but my curiosity got the best of me and, to my relief, they were not there. I must have run faster than normal to get back since I was out of breath when I got closer to the lodge. I arrived back a little after 5:00 a.m. and, to my surprise, one of my friends was up and studying a local map at the kitchen table. Before I had a chance to share my moose story, the cabin owner arrived to prepare our breakfast before we headed to the fishing boat.

He calmly called our attention to a black bear outside. Imagine my relief that I had missed that bear and my joy to be inside the safety of our cabin. I ran upstairs and woke everyone up so they could take their first pictures and videos of a black bear in Alaska.

While up in Gustavus, I stretched indoors and on the fishing boat but avoided running outdoors again. Together, my friends and I took a few hikes after dinner and I felt confident that my legs were ready for the San Francisco Marathon. On the way back home, we had to wait one day for our connecting flight in Juneau, Alaska. I took the opportunity to lead everyone on a long hike that lasted almost four hours. We climbed nearly 4,000 feet through the cold rain forest of Juneau to get up to an incredible panoramic view. The hike was long and it rained occasionally. We even added a half an hour to the early part of the trail since we got lost and had to backtrack. The summit was a tourist destination but, because of that, it had a tram and we rode it back down in less than five minutes. This gave me an excellent bit of cross training for the marathon.

Despite some bad dreams the night before the race, it turned out to be a good day to run the San Francisco Marathon. The mile markers were better and larger this year. All the events (marathons, two half marathons, and the 5k) had a total of 19,000 participants with approximately 5,000 running the full marathon. I remember back in 2004, there were not even 2,000 of us running the full. With better promotion of the race and the opening of the Golden Gate Bridge to the half and full marathoners, the race had become more popular every year. The temperature of 50 degrees Fahrenheit in August helped attract a lot of runners as well, not to mention the promise of spectacular views of the City.

This year, a few scenes stuck in my mind and distracted me on the run. I saw a lady lying on the ground at about mile 12; she had turned blue and the few people surrounding her were taking her pulse when I passed by. A hundred yards down the street, I tried to get a police-woman's attention to get help, but she was too busy directing traffic, so I just kept on running. At about mile 25 by AT&T Park, I spotted a runner sitting down and leaning on a volunteer. They had him covered with a jacket and were waiting for an EMT to arrive. He seemed to be in good hands though he looked dehydrated. On his face, I could see the determination of wanting to run or crawl that last mile just to finish the race, but it looked like he had used everything he had and, sadly, was done for the day.

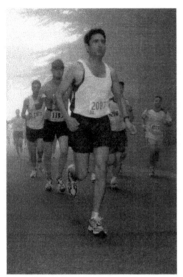

As it turned out, I needn't have worried about the boring stretch of this race. The memories of Alaska melted the dreaded miles away and sustained me throughout. That trip with friends not only took my mind off of the race when in Alaska but did second duty by distracting me during the monotonous part of the race. Before I knew it, I was back near the finish in San Francisco where I heard the roar of the spectators and spotted my wife holding our son's hand with a big smile on her face. That was a sure sign I had finished the race with a decent time.

As I became a better runner, I went back and ran this race ten more times and learned to enjoy and be present in every moment of each of those races.

Marathon Number 25
San Francisco Marathon
August 2008

Gustavus – Gustavus, formerly known as "Strawberry Point", lies on the outwash plain created by the glaciers that once filled Glacier Bay. Two hundred years ago, it was primarily a single large "beach". The native Tlingit people and others used the area for fishing, berry picking, and other similar uses. The town itself is less than one hundred years old. The first settlers arrived in 1914, but left shortly afterward. The first permanent homestead was established in 1917, when Abraham Lincoln Parker moved his family to Strawberry Point. Many Gustavus residents are descendants and relatives of the original Parker homesteaders. In 1925 the name became "Gustavus", when the U.S. Post Office required a change for its new post office, although locals continued calling it "Strawberry Point" long afterwards. The new name came from Point Gustavus at the mouth of Glacier Bay.
https://en.wikipedia.org/wiki/Gustavus,_Alaska

Juneau – Commonly known as Juneau, is the capital city of Alaska. Located in the Gastineau Channel and the Alaskan panhandle, it is a unified municipality and the second-largest city in the United States of America by area. Juneau was named the capital of Alaska in 1906, when the government of what was then the District of Alaska was moved from Sitka as dictated by the U.S. Congress in 1900.
https://en.wikipedia.org/wiki/Juneau,_Alaska

EMT - A specially trained medical technician certified to provide basic emergency services (such as cardiopulmonary resuscitation) before and during transportation to a hospital.
https://www.merriam-webster.com/dictionary/EMT

New Mexico Marathon

The 5:30 a.m. start of this race must have been due to the heat. When I looked at the weather forecast the night before the race, it showed thunderstorms for the area over the weekend and the temperature in the 70s Fahrenheit. If no rain, then it would be nice to run it. I left Saturday morning from San Jose, California and planned to return on Sunday evening after the race. Monday was Labor Day, which allowed me to get a day of rest before going back to work on Tuesday. It also meant I would be able to get back in training with my local running club a couple of days after the race. I was excited to think that, once I completed this race, I would be able to mail in my 50 States Marathon application to join the club. The club required running a marathon in at least ten states before qualifying to join.

At this point in my long-distance training I did what I called "alignment runs" the Friday before the races. Usually, this consisted of a slow two-mile run to make sure all parts of my body were functioning fine. At the end of the run in the neighborhood around my home, I got a sharp pain in my back. It ran along my right side, starting down the shoulder blade toward the lower back. The pain felt more like a muscle spasm, but sharp enough to bring me to a halt. The pain concerned me, and I thought that, if this were the race, I would have had to drop out. I walked home, took an Advil and, when I could move, got in the shower and let the hot water run on my back. In half an hour I felt better and could water the plants in our backyard and pick a few ripe figs from the tree before going to work. I called my masseuse from the office, but she did not work that day. I had hoped she would be able to make an exception for me. I knew I had to take it easy the next two days so I would be ready for the race. I thought of taking a couple of Advil with me for the run in case I needed them, although it is not a good idea to take pills in middle of a run.

We had returned from Montego Bay in Jamaica the week before. While there, I ran on the treadmill for a few days until I noticed that they had jogging on their recreation schedule at 7:30 a.m. each day. One morning, I went to the resort's office at 7:30 a.m. looking for the joggers only to find out that it was just me. They had to wake up the entertainment coordinator Duane. Poor guy showed up half asleep ten minutes later and said we were going outside for a power walk. After checking in with the front gate and hitting the pavement outside in the 80-degree Fahrenheit heat with equally high humidity, he finally figured out that I wanted to run. We started with a slow jog and picked it up half a mile down the road. By the second mile, I was gasping for air and coughing hard to clear my burning lungs as we passed a local who was enjoying his morning smoke on a dirt trail by the sea. I was glad when we got back to the resort after three or four miles and now understood why the Jamaican Olympians do so well in short distance races. As I told Duane, if you can run and train in this weather, you can run anywhere. I stayed on the treadmill in the air-conditioned gym at the resort for the remainder of the vacation and figured my one foray outside had been good training for the heat in Albuquerque, New Mexico.

I got into Albuquerque Saturday afternoon and waited with a few runners outside of the airport for the shuttle to the Best Western Hotel. After an hour the shuttle arrived and, since there was not enough room in the small shuttle, a couple of runners were left behind. I checked into the hotel when I arrived, then walked a block away over to the Hotel Albuquerque where the race expo was held. While I waited for the pedestrian light to change, I noticed that the pedestrian does not have the right of way in this town. This turned out to be a valuable lesson.

After the expo, I had lunch about three in the afternoon. My stomach had been upset because of the meal with friends the night before, plus a lack of sleep. The tacos on the menu looked good at the hotel's restaurant, but I was not going to take a chance, so I settled for a plain meal. Later I learned that was a bad choice too. The hotel had a pasta feed for the runners at 5:00 p.m., but the thought of food made me even sicker to my stomach. I decided to take a walk to the Old Town and get a souvenir for our boys. My suspicion that the pedestrians had no right of way was quickly confirmed as cars started making their right turns when it was my turn to cross the street with the walk light. I made sure to remember this pattern of driving for the next day when I would be running the race. I purchased a couple of T-shirts, and since there was not much to see, headed back to the hotel. I laid out my running gear for the next morning, set the alarm for 3:20 a.m. and went to bed by 8:00 p.m.. I woke up a few times to check on the clock and finally got up at 3:15 a.m. with my shirt soaking wet. I had turned the air conditioner off, and the room was pretty warm. I left the room by 3:45 a.m., saw a couple of runners in the lobby and then walked outside. In the nice, cool air I began walking toward the Hotel Albuquerque where I caught a bus in the parking lot to the start of the race. My stomach was doing better so I skipped breakfast.

Starting races so early in the morning, I tend to run into various people. As I walked, I saw a guy, certainly not a runner, holding his shirt and running toward me while making a strange noise. I stepped aside and let him go by, figuring he was either drunk or on some kind of drugs. When I walked into the parking lot of the hotel, I saw him again sitting at a bus stop across the street and panting pretty hard.

Once on the bus, it started raining outside. We took off in the dark with the beat of nervous hearts, the smells of Vaseline, sweat, stress, anxiety and Ben Gay filling the bus. I wished I could have opened a window, but all were locked shut. It is interesting how nervous runners like to talk loudly when being shuttled to the start of a race in an old school bus. I tried to count the number of conversations but there were just too many of them. The runner sitting next to me came from Houston and told me about their great marathon and how I should run that one next year instead of San Antonio in November. I was not in the mood to talk and just tried to rest. Luckily, a lady sitting in the next aisle picked up the conversation with him, so I no longer had to engage on the trip that took about 45 minutes to get to the start.

At the start, a guy was sitting on a folding chair playing classical guitar in the dark. A few paper lanterns shed dim light around him as we settled in the parking lot. The rain had stopped but the ground remained pretty wet. With an anticipated 400 runners to start, the lines were not too crowded for the porta-potties. The race started at 5:30 a.m. in the small town of Sandia at 5,039 feet of elevation. It took a while to adjust to the dark and make sure not to step in puddles and avoid any potholes. We were to climb 1,500 feet in the first eight miles. The silver lining of the darkness was that I could not see the climb, but the higher elevation took the best of me. I could do no better than 10-minute miles. I looked forward to mile eight where the descent would begin; by daylight we reached it. From up there, we could see the whole town of Albuquerque and the surrounding vistas. As we started the descent, the sky was overcast with a light headwind. One hot air balloon and nothing but a sleepy town hung in the distance. The drop to 1,500 feet happened in five miles and I did not mind it at all. I managed to make up for some of the lost time and kept the pace at about eight minutes per mile on the downhill. Somewhere around mile 11 or 12, I even logged a 7:45 minute per mile with the steepness of the descent. I did not want it to end, but around mile 13 we leveled off and were in the city streets before entering the bike trail of a park for the next four to five miles. Around mile 17 or 18, we encountered a few bicyclists in the park. We had to share the narrow bike trail with them, which made the run a little more challenging and interesting on a long stretch of a flat trail. We finally got back to the city streets and stayed as far away as possible from the cars that were speeding despite the presence of the traffic police. With the temperature in the mid 80s Fahrenheit , we were fortunate for the overcast sky; it would have been more challenging to run if the sun had been out. However, the heat was not anything like in Jamaica. We finished at a park across from the Atomic Museum and I felt glad that I could now become an official member of the 50 States Marathon Club.

The sweat bags were laid on the side of the street at the finish and food tables were set up inside the park. A massage after the race would have felt good, but the long line for one and hunger kept me from waiting. Before leaving, I watched young girls dressed in Mexican folkloric costumes dancing on the basketball court while I ate a banana and a small piece of bagel. I cheered the runners as I walked the racecourse back toward the hotel.

I took a shower and caught the next shuttle to the airport in the hopes of catching an earlier flight home. The friendly lady at the airline counter informed me that I had to pay an additional fee to change my flight. With the wind and rain picking up after the race and an approaching storm in the forecast, I did not want to take a chance on getting stranded. I gladly paid the fee and appreciated having the next day off to rest and recuperate. I am happy to report that my back spasm from two days prior had not bothered me at all during the race.

Marathon Number 26
New Mexico Marathon
Albuquerque, New Mexico
August 2008

Sweat Bags - Basically, volunteers will be manning a tent near the finish line/registration where runners will "check" their sweats. Volunteers will give runners a plastic bag where they can keep their sweats and will write their bib number on the plastic bag. After the race, runners come to claim their bag.
http://daviskeyclub.weebly.com/the-buzz/sweat-check-what-is-it

15 Minutes of Fame

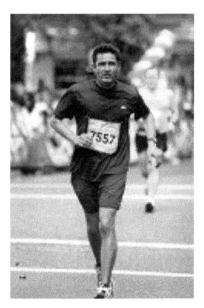

My goal of running a marathon a month for the entire 2008 came closer when my wife and I left home at 5:40 a.m. on the last Sunday of October for the Metro Silicon Valley Marathon in downtown San Jose, California. I felt good that this race would be fast and I hoped for a safe finish. I had to cancel running the Denver marathon scheduled for the prior weekend due to a recurring benign positional vertigo and this race replaced it. As we left the house, I thought that something interesting must happen sooner or later in one of these marathons.

Driving downtown, I remembered the "Early Start" option that I had read about in the race instruction. Both the marathon and half marathon were scheduled to start at 7:00 a.m. so I figured, if the race organizers allowed me to start the race early, I would avoid the rising temperatures later in the day and have an extra hour to finish. We arrived at the start line at 5:55 a.m. and I registered for the "Early Start". There was just enough time for the volunteer in charge to take my bib numbers before I stepped into the street at 6:00 a.m. and heard "GO"!

A small group of us started the race early and I took off fast. Half a mile into the dark I looked back to see no one in sight. I moved forward by following the arrows painted on the pavement. I enjoyed the cool morning air and serenity of darkness but kept being caught in the headlights of fast-moving cars going by me too closely. It confused and startled me that no traffic control was in place for those doing the "Early Start" of this race. It seemed to me the route was not designed for these runners. For many years, I trained on Los Gatos Creek Trail, which comprised part of the marathon. This came in handy when I hit the familiar trail, grateful that the shadows of feral cats now provided the only suspense in the darkness.

At the first aid station, volunteers were still setting up their tent. I was early and they were not prepared for me. They congratulated me for being in first place and hustled to fill up my water bottle. Eventually, I learned to call out "early start" before approaching the water stops so they would be prepared. At dawn's light, I arrived to the third aid station at Vasona Park in Los Gatos and received cheers from the volunteers. I still held the lead and arrived first at that station. As they cheered, I gladly played the part of the lead runner. However, when I left the aid station, I heard a volunteer say, "He must have been an Early Start, there is no way." I smiled as I picked up the pace.

The turn-around point at the track of Los Gatos High School was a lonely experience. The look of a sleepy person on the bleachers confirmed the fact that no one cared about a runner being out there so early in the morning. Even the volunteers were surprised to see me. After leaving the high school, I walked up the hill on Kennedy Street. By then I hoped for an Elite to catch up so I could stop being in the lead. On the return, I felt happy to see some orange cones set up on Blossom Hill Road. It made me excited to be the first one back into the trail; the Elites could wait.

At first, the Elite runners heading to the halfway point refused to acknowledge my presence. Soon enough, they cleared the way for me. The sound of their cheers made me imagine myself in the role of the lead runner. Their words of encouragement invigorated me so much that I picked up my pace and the miles started to melt away. My right knee begged me to stop, but how could I ruin my 15 minutes of fame? Cheers from the runners on the other side of the trail going toward the turn-around at the high school followed me all the way to mile 17 before the actual lead runner passed me following a bicycle. The bicycle acted as the lead vehicle, clearing the way for the first-place runner. Now I became more determined to be in second place.

That dream did not last long as the Elites started passing me in groups. I had been running fast by then and got very tired. Relief set in when I glimpsed the aid tent of my running club, San Jose Fit, in Campbell Park. I stopped. Seeing a friend at the aid station proved to be a blessing. I held an iced sponge to my neck and, although I felt exhaustion, retained my manners and remarked on how nice it was to see her. As I left that aid station, I realized that I had used everything I had and still had another 10 kilometers to go.

At that point my time was 3:37. I do not know why but my brain kept on subtracting an hour. When I reached mile 21, I thought my time was 2:27. I felt a tap on my shoulder and my friend from the aid station appeared, like a concerned angel. She was a runner and had left her post at the aid station to follow me. The expression on my face must have shown my pain because she started giving me instructions. I just followed her directions and lay down on someone's front lawn while she stretched my legs for what seemed like an eternity. As my tired body relaxed on the grass, my inner timer must have stopped also. My happy brain refused to recognize it until mile 25.

In previous races, taking electrolytes at the mile marker 25 used to bring me back to earth, but not this time. This was not like the other marathons. I figure I walked most of the last five miles with a mild vertigo. The overexertion may have caused the dizzy sensation I experienced. By the time I recognized that I was close to the finish line, I did something similar to running in the last mile. My wife gave me a high five with a concerned look when I crossed the finish line. I knew I must not have looked too well. The finish line clock showed 3:45 and my brain was still subtracting an hour due to my early start. I did the math correctly after the race, I should have added an hour since I started early. My time was 4:45. Something interesting happened that day, I had my 15 minutes of fame.

Marathon Number 28
Silicon Valley Marathon
San Jose, CA
October 2008

Benign Positional Vertigo - Benign positional vertigo (BPV) is the most common cause of vertigo, the sensation of spinning or swaying. It causes a sudden sensation of spinning, or like your head is spinning from the inside.
https://www.healthline.com/health/benign-positional-vertigo

Aid Station - At endurance races like marathons or bicycle racing events, aid stations are established along the race route to provide supplies (food, water, and repair equipment) to participants
https://en.wikipedia.org/wiki/Aid_station#:~:text=At%20endurance%20races%20like%20 marathons,and%20repair%20equipment)%20to%20participants.&text=Depending%20 on%20the%20length%20of,supplies%20will%20also%20be%20available.

Elite Runner - Without fail, elite runners are very close to 180 steps per minute. The cadence of average runners, on the other hand, can vary significantly. It is not uncommon for the cadence of an average runner to be less than 160 steps per minute, and sometimes as low as 140.
https://panthersportsmedicine.com/blog/3-differences-between-elite-runners-and-aver-age-runners/

Cadence - In running, cadence is often defined as the total number of steps you take per minute. One easy way to measure your cadence for running is to count the times your feet hit the ground in 60 seconds. ... Cadence is one of the two factors that make up a runner's speed
https://www.polar.com/blog/what-is-running-cadence/#:~:text=In%20running%2C%20 cadence%20is%20often,the%20ground%20in%2060%20seconds.&text=Cadence%20is%20 one%20of%20the,make%20up%20a%20runner's%20speed

Pace - In running, pace is usually defined as the number of minutes it takes to cover a mile or kilometer. Pacing is often a critical aspect of endurance events. Some coaches advocate training at a combination of specific paces related to one's fitness in order to stimulate various physiological improvements.
https://en.wikipedia.org/wiki/Pace_(speed)#:~:text=In%20running%2C%20pace%20is%20 usually,to%20stimulate%20various%20physiological%20improvements.

Electrolytes - Electrolytes are the medium that transfers electricity throughout the body. Essentially, they're salts, just like the ones you'd consume at any meal. When you sweat, you lose electrolytes, including sodium, chloride and potassium.
https://trailrunnermag.com/nutrition/ask-the-sports-rd-what-are-electrolytes-and-how-much-do-i-reallyneed.html#:~:text=Electrolytes%20are%20the%20medium%20that,in-cluding%20sodium%2C%20chloride%20and%20potassium

Chilling in San Antonio, Texas

The Rock and Roll Marathon — not only one more state to cross off my 50 State list, but also one more adventure with unexpected experiences!

The morning of the race brought an unanticipated cold spell. In more ways than one, I had not prepared for anything that came before the start of the race. As usual, I began the day early and got to the race area two hours ahead of schedule. First challenge of the day – no space to park. I had to drive a few times between the start and finish line looking for a space; it seemed like the whole town had come. Finally, I parked my rental car at AT&T Center, the home of the San Antonio Spurs of the National Basketball Association. I was happy to have budgeted enough time this morning as I had not expected that finding a parking spot would be so challenging. I looked at my watch and saw I had plenty of time to spare. I grabbed all that I needed and headed to the shuttle that would take me to the start line. Only a few people waited for the shuttle, surprising since the parking challenge indicated otherwise.

Getting off the shuttle, I realized I only had on my running attire ready to run a race, but I had a long wait before the start, and it was cold. I had not brought any other clothing with me. I started walking around looking for things that might help take my mind off the cold air chilling me to the bone. I stopped at the Volunteer's tent where I grabbed a bagel and a banana. The tent felt good and kept me warm temporarily. Of course, I was not allowed to stay there for long, so continued walking. I managed to find a spot near a building in the hopes that it would shield me from the cold wind. As a runner, I do not store much fat in my body, so I felt the cold air even more. Soon I saw I was not the only one shivering; many other runners had failed to bring enough warm clothing as well. Too cold for me to move around and stretch, I sat on a corner, watched other runners pass by and observed how individuals coped with the cold situation that morning.

A most interesting scene caught my attention, something that described human behavior in circumstances like this very well. A few runners had congregated around generators powering the lights. I thought perhaps the light's heat helped them stay warm but, after paying more attention, it appeared they were hovering over the generator's exhaust fan. What an idea! I left my corner and walked toward one of the generators to test the effectiveness of the heat from the exhaust. At the time I thought, if the heat were not enough, at least being with other people would help me warm up.

Walking closer to the generator's fan, I noticed the circle of people around the exhaust began huddling closer to one other. Now I thought, "that is how working together works." I proudly looked forward to being a part of keeping others warm and eagerly went to join the tight circle. Reality sunk in when I noticed they used the tightness in an attempt to discourage any newcomers from entering in. I decided this collective effort was not pre-planned; the cold simply had to have dictated their reaction. I forgot all about the cold while I observed the group demonstrate the same behavior when others approached seeking warmth. I never could get close enough to find out how much warmth emanated from the exhaust fan. I could hear one runner say that the fumes from the exhaust would not be beneficial for the run. Not too many people noticed the comment and, if they did, they were too cold to move.

Walking away from the stingy generator crowd, I glanced at my watch to see that I still had a lot of time before the start of the race. I began looking around for a new way to stay warm and a space across from me caught my eye. In a fenced area about 400 square feet, a crowd of runners gathered under four gas-burning heaters, one on each corner. From afar they looked like penguins huddled together for warmth. However, I sensed something different about this group of people in a circle around the heat. When I approached the fenced area, my optimistic brain thought, "This is what these races are all about, humans caring for each other." To me, this behavior represented a highlight of the race because it defined an aspect of human behavior with respect to how we care for one another when needed. Unfortunately, I discovered the opposite to be true; they only cared about themselves. I assumed these people must have paid a special fee in order to be part of such a privileged group and enjoy the heat while waiting for the race to start. Naturally, they were the envy of the crowd. As I imagined the warmth of the heaters, I noticed other runners getting attracted to the heaters and walking toward the fenced area. However, once they got closer, the same behavior occurred similar to the group at the exhaust fans of the light generators. The crowd inside rejected them with an unwelcome looks at a subconscious level. Granted, they also had the advantage of being separated by a temporary plastic fence. While I watched different runners approaching the fenced area and getting rejected, I began to ponder the reason for their rejection. Were they rejected because they had not paid the fee and were not entitled to the heat? Or was it that they did not share the same rank because they had not arrived to the fenced area at the right time?

These observations helped me forget about the cold until the race started. The behavior I witnessed did not leave my mind. When I thought more about it during the race, I realized that, as humans, we have a long way to go before we are compassionate enough to want to take care of one another. Even with all the technology at our disposal, we still need to outgrow the stage of struggle for survival. In addition, my observations confirmed the validity of the studies done on humans when, given a certain rank considered to be above others, their behavior changes to fit that rank.

I find it helpful during these long runs to have distractions along the way. It pleased me to have the rest of the race to think about what I had seen during the cold morning wait. Also, the sounds of rock bands singing their lungs out filled the miles while the cheerleaders from various high schools in San Antonio competed for our attention throughout the course. I am sure at least one band played for every mile of the race.

At one point in the race, I saw a gurney being pushed by paramedics with a defibrillator sitting on top of it. Not a good sight to see during a race. It took me back to earlier that morning when someone had said the fumes of the light generators were not good for runners, yet none moved away from them. I hoped that injury was not bad.

Around mile 14, I started to feel the weight of the marathons I had been running that year. I slowed down drastically by mile 24. No matter, because I realized that when I finish this one, I would be that much closer to my goal of running one marathon a month for an entire year.

The day had gotten warmer and I had not even noticed because there were enough other things that kept me warm. Once I finished, I discovered that 33,000 participants had started the inaugural Rock and Roll Marathon of San Antonio with me. Among them, about 18,000 finished the half and close to 8,000 finished the full marathon. Funny to think these same people, who did not want to share the heat of the light generators or the gas heaters, all had no problem running the race together.

Marathon Number 29
Rock and Roll San Antonio Marathon
San Antonio, TX
November 2008

Human Behavior - is the potential and expressed capacity (mentally, physically, and socially) of human individuals or groups to respond to internal and external stimuli throughout their life.
https://en.wikipedia.org/wiki/Human_behavior#:~:text=Human%20behavior%20is%20the%20potential,external%20stimuli%20throughout%20their%20life

Eating New Orleans

My last marathon of the year was on December 7, 2008 in Las Vegas, Nevada and I took sick soon after I got back home. The kids brought home all kinds of viruses from school and, given that my immune system was compromised, I easily contracted a viral infection. I had planned to take a couple of weeks off of running and recover from all my runs in 2008, but not like this. The cold had me down and I had no choice but to rest and drink lots of fluids, based on the doctor's advice. I got better before we took our boys skiing around Christmas but, while away, not only did I catch the stomach flu from our travel companions but, to top it off, our friends' kids gave me another cold. I was pretty miserable on New Year's Day; however, I managed a short run the day before to commemorate my last run of the year. The advice nurse had prescribed cough medicine with codeine, which was no help. I got sicker as the days went by in the New Year. Finally, I paid a visit to my doctor to find out that my left lung had partially collapsed. She did not prescribe antibiotics so my immune system alone had to fight the viral infection. Given that I had a marathon coming up in February and could not run to train for it, there were a couple of stressful weeks in early January that did not help with my recovery. At last, I started getting better by the third week of January and managed to do a few runs.

A week before the race I decided not to cancel and kept my trip to New Orleans, Louisiana as planned. This decision was made due to the fact that I had signed up to run the Paris Marathon in April and I knew the New Orleans Marathon would be a good training run to help me get back into running shape. I knew that I would not be able to run strong, but committed to do my best and finish the race in a decent time.

I got to New Orleans through Denver on Friday, January 30th. After waiting for the shuttle at the airport forever, I finally arrived at my hotel by the convention center. When I checked into my room, I noticed there was a loud party going on next door. After a while, I figured that I would not be able to rest for the race so I went back to the front desk and asked for a quieter room. They sent me to the seventh floor where, apparently, no one had visited for a long time. The room had a damp, smoky kind of smell and it did not feel right. I called them with my concern and they offered to send up an air purifier. I ended up at the front desk again. This time they were nice enough to give me a suite since I had gone up and down the elevator so many times. The room was just perfect and I really did not want to leave it to go for dinner. The front desk told me about a place a few blocks away called Mulate's Cajun Restaurant that offered local food.

When I stepped outside, I remembered the shuttle driver's advice that I should not engage in conversation with the passers-by. He believed the reason tourists got in trouble in this town was because they engaged with people hanging in the street. I had a few sightings of the kind of people he had warned me about on my way to Mulate's but, overall, the town had a warm feel to it.

I found the local Bach Amber from the tap quite tasty and the seafood gumbo delicious. I surprised the lady at the bar when I ordered alligator meat, but she soon got over it and recommended the blackened version. The meat had a very different texture; nothing like the mix of chicken and squid the bartender claimed. It had a fatty texture that was chewy with a muddy aftertaste. Of course, picturing the alligator while eating it did not help, but I kept the woman behind the bar pretty amused as she watched me wash it down with a second beer. I told her that this was the second time I had eaten strange meat, the other time being in the Philippines when I ate monkey meat. Needless to say, she was grossed out when I admitted to her that I had not been aware the meat I ordered then had been that of a monkey. She and her coworker behind the bar gave me strange looks and they both shook their heads. Funny, they thought alligator meat was normal and monkey meat a taboo. Darwin's fault: if he had claimed that we were the descendants of reptiles, then we might not be eating alligators. I enjoyed the music of the live band while they played the night away, but I had to get back to the hotel for a good night's sleep. I donated to the tip jar and picked up one of their CD's to listen to later. I also called my son in San Diego, California to brag about eating alligator and he recommended that I be a tourist the next day and check out Café Du Monde in the French Quarter for beignets and Coffee Chicory.

It took me a while to find the race expo the next morning, but it was a nice walk to the Hilton Convention Center. Apparently, every hotel has its own convention center, plus another building existed called the Convention Center that occupied multiple blocks. I am sure I was not the only one lost that morning. I found nothing special about the small race expo, but appreciated how the volunteers displayed their Southern hospitality. I returned to my hotel for some reading before heading out to the French Quarter. Having read about it, and knowing the place from the programs on the Food Channel, I was curious about the Quarter. I walked by the Mississippi River and arrived at the heart of the French Quarter. A few bands played in the streets, all sounding quite good. I had to hold back on buying their CD's. All the bands had their CD's for sale while they played, a good idea for generating income since the tourists, seemed to want something for their money. After walking around and checking out the crowd, I asked a shopkeeper about the Coffee Chicory and she pointed me toward Café Du Monde. Of course, it could not be missed. I had not had coffee in over 15 years, but I tried a cup with the hot fresh beignets (the local overrated powdered sugar donuts). I picked up a can of coffee for my son when I left. I sat in the sun for a while and watched DMC Group do their break dance routine, make fun of passers-by and hustle the audience for $20.00 bills. They managed to fill their buckets by the end of the show. Their claim to fame was an appearance on TV's "America's Got Talent" the year before. Good act and great hustlers.

I took long walks and rested, then had dinner at the mall in the river walk – a fried catfish that was mostly breaded with a tiny bit of fish inside. I just could not risk any exotic food the night before the race, even though it was tempting. The morning of the race dawned uneventful. I took a walk from the hotel to the New Orleans's Superdome twelve blocks away. When I left the hotel, I noticed people waiting for cabs to get to the start line and, as I walked by a few other hotels, I noticed more of the same. It is always interesting to see runners waiting for cabs or elevators. How ironic to want to run a race but not walk to the start or not take the stairs and instead wait in line for an elevator for one flight up. To my disappointment, no music played at the start after all, this was New Orleans, but they were proud to announce the flying of a Coast Guard helicopter overhead. The race organizers had mapped out a sanitized route for us to assure that we did not witness the poverty or the devastation of Hurricane

Katrina from four years before. During the second mile of the race, we passed through the famous Bourbon Street but were only greeted by spectators hungover from the night before and cheered by bewildered prostitutes. The narrow street had been washed with soap and water and its wetness required a lot of focus to not slip and fall. I ran with the 3:20 pace group for a while before slowing down to let the 3:40 pace group pass me. Later in the race the 4:00 hour pace group left me in the dust. The lack of training since my last marathon did not allow me to do well on the course, so I decided to take it easy and enjoy the run. I stopped at most water stations, walked a few miles toward the end and talked to a few runners along the way. The highlight of the finish line was a meal of rice and red beans, which I enjoyed before taking a cab back to the hotel. The cab driver was in a hustling mood and well aware that he could take advantage of the tired runners at the end of the race. After the marathon, I appreciated having a suite with a Jacuzzi in the room – a great help for a quick recovery. From there, I got a burger at a nearby restaurant by the hotel before catching the shuttle back to the airport.

On the way to the airport I remembered that, while I walked the last miles of the race, my mind was already planning my next race. I guess I finally had gotten over my cold, flu and collapsed lung if I was feeling good enough to envision a local race before the Paris Marathon in April.

Marathon Number 31
New Orleans, Louisiana
February 2009

Beignets - a light square doughnut usually sprinkled with powdered sugar.
https://www.merriam-webster.com/dictionary/beignet

Training run – Implies running with a purpose other than fitness. Training means that you have set a specific running goal and are implementing a plan in order to achieve that goal. The running goal may be associated with a distance, a time, or both.
https://www.runnersworld.com/beginner/a20846571/can-you-explain-training-terminology/#:~:text=Many%20people%20run%20for%20a,%2C%20a%20time%2C%20or%20both

French Quarter - Also known as the Vieux Carré, is the oldest neighborhood in the city of New Orleans.
https://en.wikipedia.org/wiki/French_Quarter

Hurricane Katrina - Was a large Category 5 Atlantic *hurricane* that caused over 1,800 deaths and $125 billion in damage in August 2005, particularly in the city of New Orleans and the surrounding areas.
https://en.wikipedia.org/wiki/Hurricane_Katrina

The City of Love

Paris, France. What a wonderful place to spend a holiday with family, celebrate my birthday and run my first international marathon. It did not take much persuasion for my family to accompany me to Paris. We got there a few days before the race and celebrated my birthday with a wonderful dinner in an intimate French restaurant near the place where we were staying. We had chosen the traditional artist district (Montmartre) so that our young boys (6 and 10) would get a better sense of the art scene in Paris. Working with oils, I have done a lot of paintings through the years. Staying at the heart of the art district felt like being at home. In her college years, my wife had spent her summer vacations in Paris. She was our guide while we discovered more of the City of Love. In the days prior to the marathon, we took the opportunity to do some sightseeing and visit friends. Our boys were fascinated by the fact that people lived outside of United States, since their formal elementary school education had introduced the U.S. as being the center of the universe. They could not get enough of croissants and orange juice in Paris and made a meal of them at every given opportunity.

The large size of the race expo amazed me. I found it filled with lots of vendors and many private booths promoting other European marathons. Most volunteers spoke English and the process of picking up race bibs and shirts went pretty smoothly. Our boys occupied themselves with the play booths set up for children and a rock-climbing wall. They paid very little attention to the expo. A giant screen outside displayed the race from last year, which helped me to understand the course a little better. It was fun to hang around with other runners from all over the world and watch the well-edited video showing the elite runners passing by the major monuments. With the help of the volunteers at the expo, I learned how the Paris Metro could easily take me to the start of the race on marathon day.

I got to the race early enough to observe some of the set-up and preparation before checking my sweat bag and heading to my race corral on the Champs-Elysees. We were separated by colors on our bibs according to our finish times from qualifying marathons. Despite all the negative comments of runners from previous years, I found the race to be well organized at the start. There were plenty of pacers in each corral and prior to start, we could see the news helicopter circling overhead. Large corrals usually start in waves, with the objective being to prevent overcrowding. However, I heard from the other runners around me that in this marathon, our corral of 10,000 would all start at the same time. I tried not to think of the congestion this would create on some of the narrow streets of Paris. While we waited, I observed some of the runners throwing their extra clothing and water bottles in the middle of road with no regard for the safety of other runners. Unfortunately, this theme continued throughout the day.

The race started with the music from the "Chariots of Fire" movie soundtrack booming on the loudspeakers around us. Besides the challenge of running a marathon, we also had to navigate the streets crowded with thousands of runners while trying not to stumble on the clothing and other waste thrown onto the roads. The first five kilometers proved difficult because of the crowds of runners. We even came to halt on the narrow streets near the Bastille. With the congestion, I switched to a slow walk before the next aid station.

The water stations were 2.5 kilometers apart and stocked with wet sponges, water in plastic bottles, energy drinks, oranges, bananas, dried apricots, raisins, sultanas, sugar cubes and, in the last 10 kilometers, they supplied wine, cider, Haribo gummi candy, bread and cake. Running through these water stations became challenging since I had to navigate my way through a muddy road covered with banana and orange peels, wet and dirty sponges, bottle caps and half empty bottles of water. All of these goodies created a lot of waste and made the roads hazardous. Later in the race, we passed by aid stations that had run out of water sponges and volunteers were throwing cups of water on runners.

Besides tripping on trash, injuries also occurred simply by participants running into each other at times. When someone sustained an injury on the course, it was customary for the runners to stop and clear the way for the paramedics. Ambulances continued to pass us in a hurry with their deafening sirens, confirming there were no shortages of injuries that day.

Hundreds of spectators lined the roads along the way and the friendly ones shouted our names (from our race bibs) with an "allez!" (go!). Part of the course passed over cobblestone-lined streets that required a lot of attention. We also ran on a path that dipped down alongside the banks of River Seine. Passing by the historic landmark of the Eiffel Tower, coupled with the cool breath from the river, helped take my mind off the frustrating parts of the run. There were occasions of sunshine, however the temperature did not rise above 22 degrees centigrade (71.6 Fahrenheit). An ideal temperature for a race. We had arranged for our family meeting at a spot by the River Seine around the 26th kilometer of the race where we had walked the day before. However, I never saw them and later I learned that they showed up after I had passed by. Frustrated by the congestion on the narrow streets that forced me to walk part of the race, I felt pretty tired and discouraged. When I saw the 40-kilometer mark and heard the cheers of the crowd in the last two kilometers, my spirits lifted.

The finish area had a fairly efficient set-up that sought to avoid overcrowding. The area seemed well organized and the volunteers made sure the runners did not pick up more than their share of food so that there would be enough for all participants. After getting our food, they had us walk another half kilometer to the sweat bag area to collect our gear. Later I read that, for those runners who finished after us, it became a challenge to get through the finish area due to heavy congestion. In the sweat bag area, I tried not to watch other runners throwing up. This appeared to be a badge of honor for many who had just completed the Paris Marathon.

As much as I had hoped to see my family at the finish, I was happy they did not show up in that chaotic scene. Instead, I crammed onto an extremely crowded Metro and, after a short walk from the station, arrived at our apartment for a much-needed shower.

The Paris Marathon is now off my bucket list. I would not endeavor to run it again because of the overcrowding, the slow run times, the cobblestones and garbage-strewn streets. I had a better time just being there with my family than running the marathon.

Marathon Number 33
Paris Marathon
Marathon De Paris
April 2009

Race Bib - A piece of cloth, paper, or plastic with an identifying number that is worn by a participant in a race or contest a race bib.
https://www.merriam-webster.com/dictionary/bib#:~:text=4%20%3A%20a%20piece%20of%20cloth,or%20contest%20a%20race%20bib

Pacer: Generally, a pacer is an experienced runner that runs at a set speed in a race, typically a long-distance event. This helps you finish at your desired time. You don't have to think too hard about your pace.
https://www.canaanvalleyhalfmarathon.com/why-should-you-use-a-pacer-for-running/#:~:text=Generally%2C%20a%20pacer%20is%20an,too%20hard%20about%20your%20pace

Sultanas – sometimes just called golden raisins, are golden-colored dried grapes that are made from various varieties of seedless white-fleshed grapes. The skin of these fruits start off as pale yellow in color, but unlike raisins, don't darken in the same way as they dry.
https://www.thekitchn.com/whats-the-difference-between-raisins-sultanas-and-currants-223285

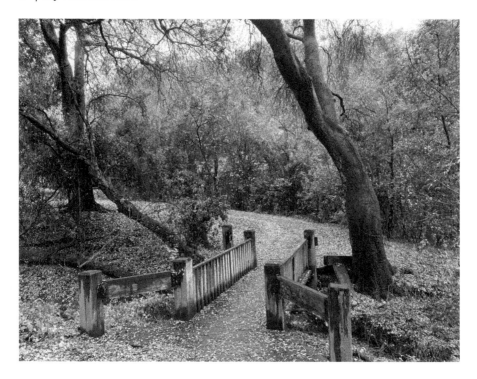

My First Trail Race

For my first trail race, I chose the 30 Kilometer (18.64 miles) distance in order to get acquainted with trail racing. Previous races had been exclusively on the road. The race web site indicated that we would run a 20 Kilometer (12.43 miles) , followed by a 10 Kilometer (6.2 miles) loop. The 20 Kilometer course would have 2,900 feet of elevation gain, but the site did not mention if the elevation loss would be the same. I did not read about the elevation gain for the 10 Kilometer loop prior to the start of the race.

When I took the exit toward Redwood Regional Park in Oakland, California on the morning of the race in 2009, I found myself in the neighborhood where I went to the English Language Institute nearly 31 years ago. The Institute is now called Holy Names University. I felt good to be back in the old neighborhood for a trail run. The weather cooperated and, as a result of the recent California drought, the park and trail were dry. At the start we learned that most people were running the 10 Kilometer race, a few opted for the 50 Kilometer and the rest of us were running the 30 Kilometer distance.

The first climb challenged me as the ascent went straight up from the start. I had to walk up most of it, although there were a lot of young runners who ran it. Not long after the start, a guy tripped on a rock and took a bad fall in front of me. When I passed him and asked if he were okay, he said he was fine, that this was a "tuck and roll" and he would probably experience another one before the finish of the race. "What a self-fulfilling prophecy," I thought.

The aid station came at 8.5 kilometers, followed by another climb up before leveling off and going toward the east ridge of the park. Once there, I encountered a short, forested trail shrouded in a fog that provided a welcoming mist. The scenery was breathtaking; however, its beauty could not distract me. I had to stay focused and look out for tree roots, rocks, boulders and other obstacles on the trail in order to be assured of a safe run. In theory that would have worked; in practice, this proved difficult. On the way down the east side about 15 kilometers into the race, I became consumed by the allure of nature's bounty as I ran along a narrow ridge with a drop of 1,000 feet. I remember enjoying the speed of the downhill right before I landed flat on my face, screaming with pain. It took a while to catch my breath and be able to get up and assess the damage. Upon examination, the external injuries included splinters in both hands and knees burning due to bruising and bleeding. I could not see my face. But more than the physical pain was the reality of rejoining the course and finishing the race with injuries. I tried very hard to understand how I fell but could not figure it out. I walked down the hill until another runner passed by. I stopped her while I stepped aside from the trail and asked her how I looked. She said fine, then came in for a closer look and told me the bleeding was not too bad. I limped and managed to get to the next aid station located near the beginning of the 10 Kilometer loop trail. I asked for water and washed my wounds. A volunteer fixed the strap of my water bottle that had come loose. I washed the bottle, filled it with water and took off toward the 10 Kilometer loop. The looks of passing runners testified to my bleeding body and the amount of dirt painted on my clothing.

When I saw the climb a kilometer into the trail, I stopped my painful jog and walked. I thought that the race director had quite a sense of humor to be designing such a tough course. I briefly wondered if I should just return to the aid station and call off the race. But quitting was not an option; I had to finish the race. So I toughed it out and climbed about 1,500 feet while listening to crackling sounds from my knees. I found a stick on the side of the trail and used it to help me with the climb. Many times, I had to step aside so other runners behind me could pass. Most were supportive and offered help, but I told them I was fine. One runner's discouraging words conveyed what would be a pain-filled experience on the climb down. She did not exaggerate as I came upon the descent. Somewhere toward the finish on the narrow trail, a volunteer search and rescue patrol stopped me to help. He carried a big pack on his back, put it down and offered to clean and fix up my wounds. I refused, but asked for water since my supply was short. It felt like forever before he fished a bottle of water out of his backpack and filled my water bottle. As I left, I heard him on his CB Radio calling someone with my bib number. It was, indeed, agonizing to walk down the drop since I feared another fall. With shaky knees, I tripped a couple of times but stayed upright while the other runners passed me by. Earlier, I had told the search and rescue man that my feelings hurt more than my physical injuries.

I happily reached the flat ground near the end, with the expectation of getting some help now that I had finished. No one paid attention to me because the race director and volunteers were consumed by the story of a guy who had just finished the 50 Kilometer race with a torn shirt. They reveled in his account of how his iPod had flown out of his hand on a downhill but he had not gone after it. I got some soup and sat down while listening to more of the runner's adventures on the course that day. I got up, asked a volunteer for ointment and bandages and limped toward my car. I sat in the back of the car fixing my knees when a guy who had just finished the race told me that I was lucky not to have broken any limbs. That is when I realized that trail runners are a different breed, I wanted to be one of them. This was my first trail race.

30k Trail Run
Redwood Regional Park
Oakland, California
September 2009

Tuck and Roll - basically means to do a somersault.
https://www.italki.com/post/question-202231?hl=en

Self-fulfilling prophecy - Is a prediction that causes itself to be true due to the behavior (including the act of predicting it) of the believer. Self-fulling, here, means "brought about as a result of being foretold or talked about," while prophecy refers to the prediction.
https://www.dictionary.com/e/pop-culture/self-fulfilling-prophecy/

CB Radio – Citizens band radio (also known as CB radio), used in many countries, is a land mobile radio system, a system allowing short-distance person-to-person bidirectional voice communication between individuals, using two way radios operating on 40 channels near 27 MHz (11 m) in the high frequency (a.k.a. shortwave) band
https://en.wikipedia.org/wiki/Citizens_band_radio

iPod - The iPod is a line of portable media players and multi-purpose pocket computers designed and marketed by Apple Inc. The first version was released on October 23, 2001, about 8 1/2 months after the Macintosh version of iTunes was released. As of May 28, 2019, only the iPod Touch (7th generation) remains in production.
https://en.wikipedia.org/wiki/IPod

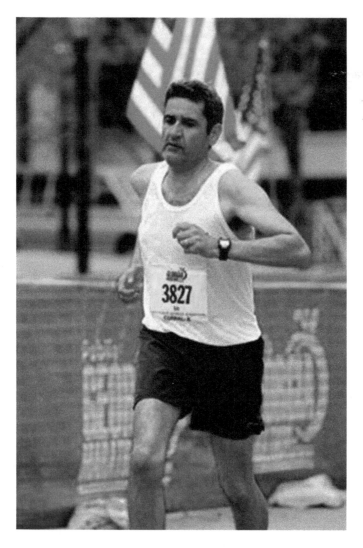

Patriot Run

To honor the troops and keep the memory of 9/11 alive, this run took place on September 11, 2009. The registration fee cost was only $25.00 (the lowest of all marathon fees I have paid so far). For an extra $9.11 you could buy a T-shirt or eat a pasta dinner. You could also run the ultra, as an official race, from noon until 9:11 p.m. The race was held in the town of Olathe, Kansas. I flew into Kansas City International the day before, picked up my little rental car and drove to Olathe. I worried about the really warm temperatures and high humidity and hoped the next day would be cooler for the run. After checking into my hotel, I planned to go to the race expo at the Salvation Army to pick up my bib and gear. The hotel desk clerk gave me the directions to get there and, considering the small size of Olathe, I discovered it was not too far away. At the expo, I picked up my number then peeked into the ballroom where they had set up tables covered with white cloths for the pre-race pasta dinner. I did not feel like sticking around, instead I ate at the BBQ place next to the hotel. I loved the food and found myself comparing the varying barbecues of Texas, Tennessee and Kansas. No doubt, barbecue played a big role in the diet of this town.

Tired from my travels, I turned in early. The next morning after breakfast I hung around the hotel before the race and did some reading. By the time I found the start of the race at Twin Trail Park, the heat had set in and I began sweating. Since the marathon consisted of 36+ loops of .75 miles around the park, smart-thinking runners had stationed their cars by the trail. Some had backed up their vehicles and popped open their trunks while organizing their supplies for the day. While waiting, I watched a runner hang a few of his hand towels on a rope under a canopy by his vehicle. Once in a while he dried his face with one. He kept on hanging and rearranging his towels, which I perceived to be a sign of nervousness before the start of the race. Some runners set up lawn chairs, the military runners from the nearby army camp sat in their tents and other runners settled in with their grills and picnic supplies for a long day under the heat and humidity of Olathe.

As predicted, the marathon started at 9:11 a.m. After a couple of laps, I found it difficult to run in the sweltering heat. Luckily, the loop around the park was flat. Later in the race, one of the local runners told me the temperature hit 82 degrees Fahrenheit with humidity over 90%. I ended up walking and running while keeping track of my laps. We had electronic chips for logging our laps and times whenever we crossed the mat located at the start/finish line of the race. When I got to my last three-lap countdown, I stopped by the trailer at the start/finish and asked them to confirm my remaining laps. To my disappointment, they told me I still had seven more laps to go. I ended up walking the last few laps in the company of a local runner who showed me his little notepad and how he had counted his laps accurately but was also told that he needed to run three more. No doubt, by then we realized a problem existed with their tracking system. When I finally completed the extra laps, I stopped by the trailer to confirm my finish and had to wait for the person in charge to update his system to validate my data. The man remained unconfident about whether their system had worked well. With that in mind, I decided to declare the race finished and I wondered whether he had given me the correct information when I had queried him the first time. Now that I am looking back, it was not that important. At the time, though, I became pretty frustrated and disappointed since the race website had assured us the accurate count of our laps would be backed up by volunteers. Those volunteers were nowhere to be found at the race. When I left the park, a few runners and walkers remained doing their laps. Some continued until 9:11 p.m. for their ultras.

As I ran, I reflected back on the activities held before the start of the race. There were flag ceremonies and a live broadcast from the troops at a US military base in Afghanistan; they had completed their own run before ours began. In fact, after we watched the live feed of soldiers running in Afghanistan, one soldier mentioned in his speech prior to the start of the race that, "He was proud that our soldiers could run in the backyard of the enemy." Participants and spectators waved flags and celebrated the ninth birthdays of two local kids born on September 11, 2001. No question about the patriotism of the folks in Olathe, Kansas. September 11th was alive and well in this part of the country, even as the United States escalated the war in Afghanistan and created a high demand for new recruits. Fort Leavenworth was close by Olathe and Army recruiters maintained a heavy presence in town. I wondered if this Patriot Run was, in fact, being sponsored by the Army as a way of recruiting new soldiers.

During the race, I had opportunities to run with some of the soldiers throughout the day. It became obvious to me that they had signed up due to the influence of 9/11. They competed with their buddies about who displayed the highest degree of patriotism. Indeed, most were convinced that they were providing an invaluable service for their country.

I also ran for a few loops behind a couple of experienced soldiers and listened to one of them tell the story of how he had been told to be aware of the young sheepherders in Afghanistan working near their makeshift military camps. He described how the young sheepherders would come by the camp to ask for food and get acquainted with the soldiers only to come back on their next visit wearing a suicide vest. He bragged about how much he had enjoyed shooting rabbits on his grandfather's farm while growing up and had no trouble using his skills to shoot any young sheepherder seen near their camp. I felt sad that these sheepherders had been reduced to the status of animals to be hunted. I had read about the never-ending wars in Afghanistan and the famine that ensued as a result of farmers fleeing their villages in search of a safe haven. I also knew that any fathers, who had not been killed in the wars or forced to join a warring faction, would have taken refuge in neighboring countries with their families. With farmers and families gone, conscripted or killed, young orphans were left to fend for themselves. As a means of survival, some of these orphans became sheepherders. A vicious cycle ensued.

On the long flight home, I recalled the scene when I checked out of the hotel. The lobby had buzzed with new recruits in their fresh uniforms. They were ready to be deployed and excited to go to a land that they knew only by name. They were so young and innocent. It caused me to reflect on my job teaching management and leadership classes at the university. This work gave me an opportunity to bond with veterans coming back from various wars, a privilege that I never took for granted. In some of my classes, where the veterans felt comfortable, they would share the physical and psychological disabilities they incurred during their wartime duties. A few would take pride in competing with classmates on the number of their injuries. A few would remain totally silent with a blank look. My concern for the quiet ones grew, because I did not know what was going through their minds while I lectured on the different styles of leadership. In private conversations, a few shared about their innocence when recruited. They admitted they joined the military while they were younger, with thoughts of serving their nation; only to find out the mission was totally different once they were on the other side of the world. I wondered how many of the new recruits I saw in Olathe would return disillusioned by their wartime experience.

I chose to run this race so I could cross off another state in my quest to run a marathon in every state in the US. But aside from running a marathon, the journey also gave me an opportunity to visit a small town in Kansas, taste their food and get to know their culture. This experience afforded me a glimpse into the definition of patriotism for the majority of the citizens living in the area. In fact, two definitions of patriotism exist in the dictionary. One describes a patriot as one who loves and supports their country. The other describes a patriot as one who loves, supports and defends their country and its interest with devotion. If I had my way, we would all simply love and support our country and that would be enough.

Marathon Number 36
Patriot Run, Olathe, Kansas
September 11, 2009

Olathe - Is the county seat of Johnson County, Kansas, United States. It is the fourth-most populous city in the Kansas City metropolitan area and Kansas, with a 2010 population of 125,872. By 2019, the Census Bureau estimated Olathe's population had grown to 140,545.
https://en.wikipedia.org/wiki/Olathe,_Kansas

Flag Ceremony - A flag ceremony honors the American flag as the symbol of our country and all the hopes, dreams, and people it represents. If your group includes girls from other countries, they can honor their flags, too, and conduct an international flag ceremony. Flag ceremonies may be used for opening or closing meetings.
https://www.gswcf.org/content/dam/wcf-images/pdf-forms/Flag-Ceremony.pdf

Patriot - One who loves and supports his or her country.
https://www.merriam-webster.com/dictionary/patriot

Patriot - A person who loves, supports, and defends his or her country and its interests with devotion.
https://www.dictionary.com/browse/patriot

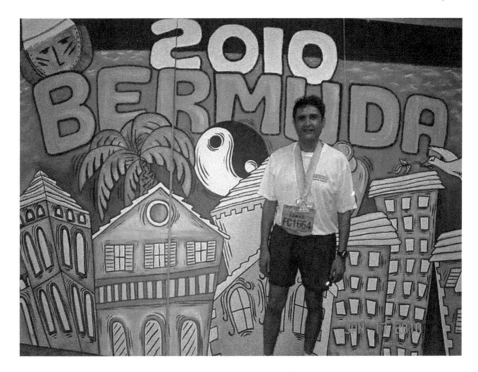

The Pink Sand

A small bottle of pink sand from Bermuda sat on my desk at work for over three decades. Back in the 80's, my boss had taken a vacation there and brought back the pink sand as a souvenir for me. He told me that I would enjoy visiting what he called the "piece of rock" in the Atlantic Ocean. After taking up distance running in 2002, the Bermuda Triangle Challenge made my bucket list. Eight years later, the idea of running the Challenge became a good reason to finally take a trip to Bermuda. The Challenge is so named because it consists of three races in three consecutive days – a fast mile on the first day, a 10-kilometer race on the second day, and a half or a full marathon on the third day.

After work in January of 2010, my wife rushed me to the airport for a red-eye flight to New York. I laid over in the early morning at JFK and then took another short flight to the island. From up above, Bermuda appeared as a huge rock amidst the Atlantic Ocean. In fact, its 21 square miles of volcanic rock can be dated back a couple of million years. Once the customs agent at the airport found out I was on the island for the Challenge, he proceeded to tell me his running stories while I watched the line behind me growing. He was not fazed with the frustration of people in line and continued to tell me that he had knee injuries and could no longer run. Once officials learn that you are a runner, this type of interaction happens to be a common experience at airports before and after the races. I do not have much choice except to nod and show interest in their stories. On the bright side, it provides an opportunity to connect with them through a common experience and see them as human rather than stoned-faced officials in a uniform. As I politely interrupted him to say good-bye, he told me that the Grotto Bay Beach Resort where I would be staying was just a hop away from the airport and quite nice.

After I checked in, the hotel clerk told me to take bus number 10 or 11 to Hamilton Resort to get to the expo that afternoon. The resort could be found in the town of Hamilton, the capitol city of Bermuda. The one-mile run was scheduled for that evening at 6:30 p.m. in Hamilton and I planned to stick around after the expo to run it. As I set out, I discovered that the roads were narrow, and it took a while to figure out how to cross the street as vehicles drove on the "wrong" side of the road. Being a British territory, the Bermudians drive by the same rules as the Brits – with the driver's seat on the right-hand side of the vehicles. I took the wrong bus and the hour or so ride to the Hamilton Resort on the other side of the island took more than two hours. However, I got to see the residential neighborhoods and, at times, shared the bus with noisy school kids as they crowded on. I found the locals to be friendly and courteous.

The no-frills expo greeted me with confused volunteers and long lines. Most T-shirt sizes were gone by the time I arrived, so I grabbed what was available. I did not see any "sweat checks" at the mile's start in Hamilton, but they directed me to where the school kids would be changing so I could leave my belongings there while running the mile of the Challenge. Excitement filled the air. It looked as if everyone on the island had come out to root for us. Cheering spectators lined up along Front Street and other people yelled from balconies. Obviously, this race meant serious business in Bermuda. They had races for the elementary schools, middle schools, high schools, local Bermudians and then the elites. Every runner had to qualify to run the mile, except those of us running the Bermuda Triangle Challenge.

Darkness began to set in when the race started. They had us in small groups in race corrals so that we did not run into each other. Being part of the Challenge, we were treated like celebrities and were given the priority to start first. Once given the go, our competitive small group took two sharp turns, and then looped up the street that had a pretty good climb. All the while we could hear the roar of the crowd. The race gave me a good introduction to the hills of Bermuda. I did not stay for the kids, Bermudians or Elite races. Later I learned they were delightful to watch. As soon as I finished with my 7:44 minute mile and, frustrated with my slow start, I went right to the bus station to get back to the Grotto Bay Beach Resort.

While waiting for the bus, I met a doctor from Colorado who was also running the Bermuda Triangle Challenge. In our conversations about running and recovery, I learned the best recovery for running is sleep. Her valuable advice would later help me be able to run multiple marathons on consecutive days and eventually get into running ultras. She also told me to learn how to listen to my body, feed it with the fuel it craves throughout my training and races, and be grateful for the gift of movement. To learn the skills of listening to my body and be present, I used what I mastered in my Tai-Chi classes. The practice of Qigong and Tai-Chi provided a natural transition into meditative running and a newfound connection to the energy of earth while walking and running. When connected to that energy, I become like a fish who does not see or feel the water they swim in, or the bird that glides through the air naturally without thinking of flying.

The next morning, I rode in a taxi with other runners from the resort to the start of our 10-kilometer race near the National Stadium. Once there, I did not feel very well and had a bit of motion sickness that did not help me in the first half of the race. Despite the hilly 10-kilometer, I finished in under an hour (59:06), then enjoyed cheering other runners as they came through the finish.

Although showers had been forecast, we enjoyed the sun and a cool breath of air. Clouds formed only in the afternoon while I took it easy at the resort. I went by the beach to take a closer look at the pink sand and swam in the warm ocean. I also discovered an ancient cave by the resort and, as tempting as it might have been to swim in the waters of the cave, I felt it would have been unsafe since I was the only one in that massive cave. I spent the rest of the afternoon in my room resting and reading. The resort had a system of saving and using the rainwater; that explained the cloudy water from the sink and shower. There were clear instructions in the room not to drink the tap water. A restaurant within walking distance of the resort provided a quiet dinner before a good night's sleep.

The next morning, I arose fairly early in order to catch our taxi to the start of the next race. I sat in the taxi for half an hour while the driver waited for the other passengers to join us. Unfortunately, they happened to board a different taxi and a fierce argument broke out between the drivers over their passengers. Instead of the anticipated six passengers, three of us split the fare to the start in Hamilton. I realized that our cab driver was not as nice as he had appeared the day before, so I told him that I would be taking the bus back after the race. The other two passengers did the same. The driver did not take the news well, but there was no time to argue.

At a school near the start of the race in Hamilton, I met a couple of elite local runners who told me their ghost stories about the race-course, which I did not care to hear. They also invited me for a fourth day of racing at the National Stadium, but I politely turned them down. After chatting with the local runners and stretching a bit, I went to the start and found out the majority of the participants were only running the half marathon. Two loops of the same course made up the marathon. The first half went pretty well, the weather cooper-ated and the picturesque scenery on the north shore provided a good diversion. Having the roads closed to traffic for the first loop was a blessing; however, after the half marathoners passed through, they opened up the second loop to traffic. With no shoulders or sidewalks, it proved to be a nerve-wracking experience to run with cars and buses coming up from behind. Once a car brushed against me and another time, I felt one passing too close. Later at the awards dinner, I found out that other runners had similar experiences. A lady caught up with me at mile 18 and we paced each other to the finish. She got a trophy for third place in her age group. At the halfway point of the race, I ran with Bart Yasoo, one of the writers for Running World Magazine.

We had a short chat about his book before he took off at mile 14. He finished ahead of me and slapped me a high five as I came toward the finish. That gave me a boost when I went through the finish line.

Our three days' results were combined, and overall winners were announced at the award ceremonies that evening. I found the doctor from Colorado and thanked her for her advice. When I was leaving the resort for the airport the next day, the wind picked up and a storm came to the island. How fortuitous we had missed the wind and rains during the past three days of racing. On my ride to the airport, my thoughts were with the elite runners of the island who were competing at the National Stadium that day.

Now, when I admire my small bottle of pink Bermuda sand, I can bring up all the sights, smells and sounds of my own journey there. I found the "rock" enticing and look forward to going back with my family for a vacation where we can relax and experience the ambiance, food and culture. No running needs be involved.

Marathon Number 38
Bermuda Triangle Challenge
Bermuda
January 15 to 17, 2010

Sweat Checks – Basically, volunteers will be manning a tent near the finish line/registration where runners will "check" their sweats. Volunteers will give runners a plastic bag where they can keep their sweats and will write their bib number on the plastic bag. After the race, runners come to claim their bag.
http://daviskeyclub.weebly.com/the-buzz/sweat-check-what-is-it#:~:text=Basically%2C%20volunteers%20will%20be%20manning,come%20to%20claim%20their%20bag.

Corrals - are supposed to sort runners into appropriate pace groups, especially at large races. They help to manage the flow of runners and guarantee that everyone moves forward at the same speed, without roadblocks. Often this requires runners to either estimate or provide proof of a previous finish time.
https://www.podiumrunner.com/training/choose-right-race-corral/#:~:text=Corrals%20are%20supposed%20to%20sort,of%20a%20previous%20finish%20time

There is always another race

The Boston Marathon is considered by most runners to be the crown jewel in the U.S. marathon circuit. There are certainly bigger, faster and more scenic races in the US, but running Boston is a badge of honor among runners. From the start of the race in Hopkinton, Massachusetts to the finish line by Copley Square in Boston, the spectators lining the streets understand the running culture. Given that there are half a million people cheering along the way is an indication of a crowd that appreciates what the runners seek to accomplish. Could it also be that they value the contributions of 27,000 runners to their economy, especially during times of recession?

I had trained well for this race and focused on the demands I would need from my body on race day. I followed a training schedule for six months prior to the race, paid close attention to my diet and made sure not to miss my core strengthening classes. After all, this was Boston Marathon and I intended to build the requisite fitness to achieve a personal record on race day.

Six days before the race, I broke one of my ribs in the core class. While lying on the cement floor doing the last set of leg raises toward the end of class, the instructor (who is a good friend) pressed on my ribs to make sure I was working from the core. The combination of the timing of the strong push, the hard surface and the leg raise caused a cracking sound. I lost my breath. As I lay with the wind knocked out of me, the instructor panicked and tried to raise me off the ground so I could breathe. With the excruciating pain, all I thought about in that moment was running the Boston Marathon in less than a week. After regaining my breath, I struggled to drive home and did my best to hide the pain from my family. I rested the next few days and did not run, while my wife shook her head and told me she hoped I would defer the race to the next year. She also knew of my stubbornness; once the goal is set, it is accomplished.

After a few days of rest and painful drives to work, I left home for a short run early Friday morning before my flight to Boston later that evening. Dragging myself to the trail, I convinced myself that I could actually run. The first few steps proved me wrong and, the more

I tried running, the harder it became to pick up my legs. I had no choice but to stop the struggle and report to the emergency room at Kaiser Hospital to find out the extent of the damage. My main concern revolved around whether the broken rib could possibly puncture my lung during the marathon. As I drove myself to the hospital, I decided that canceling Boston was not an option. I had gotten a coveted entry into the Boston Marathon and trained well for the race. The X-rays were inconclusive and required the review of a radiologist, but I did not have the time to wait. The emergency room doctor advised me not to run at all and take it easy for the next few weeks so that the fracture could heal. I asked her to listen to my lungs to make sure they had not been damaged and then requested some strong painkillers. Once she knew that she could not talk me out of going to Boston, she described the sensation of a collapsed lung so I might identify the signs if it happened to me. She further instructed me to immediately ask for help should my lung collapse during the race.

Thankfully, that evening I slept all the way to Boston because I took a strong painkiller prior to my flight departure. After I checked into the hotel in the early morning and had a short rest, I tried to walk to a race sponsored breakfast nearby. Just taking a few steps outside of the hotel turned out to be very painful since I could not catch my breath. I ended up returning to the hotel and requesting a cab. I stood in the back of the room at the breakfast, as sitting was not an option with a broken rib. As part of the ceremonies, the sponsors kept giving each other awards for their so-called charitable contributions and I felt more pain as time went by. I finally got bored with the meaningless awards ceremony and took off for the expo. I did not spend too much time there, just picked up my packet and a couple of souvenir race t-shirts for my boys before going back to the hotel in the pouring rain. I tried to run back to the hotel, but my broken rib made it impossible, so I just walked back and got soaking wet.

Admittedly, I became increasingly worried, since the marathon was the next day. I knew going for a fast finish would not be possible, so I focused on how to make the cut-off time while running with injury. I stopped at a convenience store and picked up water, Gatorade and a small bottle of Tylenol. I got a slice of pizza from a small restaurant next to the hotel, ate in my room, swallowed another painkiller, then took a nap. Later that evening, I called the hospital's advice nurse in California about my rib. She said it would be best not to run the race. She reviewed the collapsed lung symptoms with me and tried to convince me that I could run the race next year. I ignored her advice, got all my gear ready for the next day and went back to sleep.

At 5:00 a.m. race day I applied a non-prescription large pain relief patch over the broken rib and walked to the Westin Hotel from Park Plaza to catch a shuttle to the start of the race in Hopkinton. On my way, I picked up a bagel and a cup of tea from a nearby shop. While waiting in line for the shuttle, the heat of the pain relief patch was burning my skin. After a while, I felt better, but I was still trying to figure out how to run the race with my broken rib. A sunglass salesman from Canada sat next to me in the shuttle and told stories about all his injuries through the years. After hearing about my broken rib, he recommended that I take 500 milligrams of Tylenol a half an hour before the start of the race and then take another at around mile 13. I was hesitant about taking medication before the race, but the stabbing pain and the fear of not being able to run convinced me to follow his advice. I had the small bottle of Tylenol with me and I took one pill with my tea before we were dropped off near the start line of the race.

I found walking to the start, while being slightly medicated, an interesting experience. If it were not for the huge crowd around me, I may have had difficulty navigating my way to the start. On a follow up visit to my doctor after the race where he heard about the medication I took, he called me a "medicine novice" for taking Tylenol to calm the pain of a broken rib. My strategy for the race had changed at the start line, I decided to run as much as I could before finding my pace. I ran the first ten miles slowly due to excruciating pain and the challenge of breathing. Around mile eleven, I switched to a walk/slow run combination. My goal remained to finish the race before the six-hour cut-off so I could get my medal and my name in the Boston Globe newspaper. What a humbling goal; I never had to worry about cut-off times in prior marathons. Despite the pain, I enjoyed the crowd's support, especially the roar of the Wellesley College girls along the way holding signs saying "Kiss Me".

I arrived in Boston with plenty of time left before the cut-off, a huge relief for me. Some challenging moments arose in the final miles due to pain and exhaustion. I managed to finish, received my medal and saw my name published in the Boston Globe.

A few days after the race, I went to see my own doctor since the radiologist had never contacted me. Reviewing the x-rays, we could clearly see the fracture on the bottom left rib. Attached was the radiologist's note confirming it, dated from Friday afternoon when I had left the hospital. No one had bothered to get back to me, not that it would have made any difference. My own doctor also advised me to take it easy, allow the rib to heal and not run my next marathon the following month. I ran a local four-mile race with my boys six days after Boston and felt pretty good.

Since I survived running the Boston Marathon with a broken rib, nothing could stop me from continuing to run several marathons while my rib healed. Considering the risks, I do not recommend running with such injuries.

Marathon Number 41
Boston, Massachusetts
April 2010

Personal Record - A personal record or personal best (frequently abbreviated to PR or PB) is an individual's best performance in a given sporting discipline. It is most commonly found in athletic sports, such as track and field, other forms of running, swimming and weightlifting. https://en.wikipedia.org/wiki/Personal_record#:~:text=A%20personal%20record%20or%20 personal,of%20running%2C%20swimming%20and%20weightlifting.

Leg raise - The leg raise is a strength training exercise which targets the iliopsoas (the anterior hip flexors). Because the abdominal muscles are used isometrically to stabilize the body during the motion, leg raises are also often used to strengthen the rectus abdominis muscle and the internal and external oblique muscles. https://en.wikipedia.org/wiki/Leg_raise

Collapsed lung symptoms - Symptoms of collapsed lung include sharp, stabbing chest pain that worsens on breathing or with deep inhalation that often radiates to the shoulder and or back; and a dry, hacking cough. In severe cases a person may go into shock, which is a life-threatening condition that requires immediate medical treatment. https://www.emedicinehealth.com/collapsed_lung/article_em.htm

Pain relief patch - A transdermal analgesic or pain relief patch is a medicated adhesive patch used to relieve minor to severe pain. There are two primary types of analgesic patches: patches containing counterirritants, which are used to treat mild to moderate pain, and patches containing fentanyl, a narcotic used to relieve moderate to severe pain in opioid-tolerant patients. https://en.wikipedia.org/wiki/Transdermal_analgesic_patch

The Desert

I grew up in Shahrud, Iran, located in the Damghan basin, a sub-basin of the Kavir basin that contains the Great Salt Desert. From the north, Shahrud is surrounded by the Alborz mountains and from the south by the arid salty deserts. At around 4,500 feet above sea level, the summers are hot and dry while winters are cold and harsh. My family had fruit orchards and wheat farms near the edge of the desert. Growing up, we were told stories about people who ventured out into the desert and disappeared without a trace. Despite its beauty and calling, the stories discouraged me from wandering into the salt desert. In my teenage years I sat many hours at its edge, near our fruit orchards, reading and appreciating the silence and beauty of its utter starkness. When the opportunity came up to run a marathon in Death Valley, a childhood dream was awakened, and I signed up for the race.

At 282 feet below sea level, Death Valley is considered one of the hottest places on earth. It receives less than two inches of rain per year and the temperature rises up to 130 degrees Fahrenheit in the summer. Somehow, Native Americans inhabited the region in and around Death Valley since prehistoric times. Currently, only 300 people reside there. Pioneers named it during the winter of 1849-1850 when some of their group died there in the desert. Other pioneers thought of the place as their grave. With a few fatalities still occurring each year, Death Valley continues to live up to its name.

Even with such an inhospitable climate in the summer, each year the Badwater Ultramarathon is held in Death Valley. It is known as "the world's toughest foot race," consisting of a 135-mile course starting at 279 feet below sea level in the Badwater Basin in Death Valley and ending at an elevation of 8,360 feet at Whitney Portal, the trailhead to Mount Whitney. The race attracts some of the toughest ultrarunners in the world. Through the years, I have run ultras with those who have completed this race multiple times and they told me that it remains one of their most memorable running experiences. I never have had the desire to run the race since the extreme heat of the desert in the summer has always discouraged me. As a compromise, I decided to run the Death Valley Marathon, which took place in the month of February. I understood the desert to be cooler that time of the year and a marathon distance would give me a taste of running in Death Valley without having to contend with the brutal conditions of the Badwater Ultramarathon.

I flew to Las Vegas, Nevada on a Friday morning in February, rented a car, picked up a few cases of bottled water and drove 2.5 hours to Death Valley. Since my GPS could not locate the Ranch at Furnace Creek, I called them for directions, wrote the route on a piece of paper and hoped that I was driving in the right direction. I had read that most of the death in the valley is caused not by heat, but by speeding on the open road, resulting in single car crashes. Once I entered Death Valley National Park, I knew that I was on the right track. The road deceived me by appearing flat. Soon I learned that the hidden dips in the road could be blamed for some of the crashes. In fact, its subtle descent to below sea level made me keep a close eye on my speed. The scenery was breathtaking. I made a few stops whenever I encountered a shoulder where I could pull off and take in the vast beauty of the landscape. After checking in at the Ranch at Furnace Creek, I drove to see more of the desert in the late afternoon and stayed for the sunset on the road to Badwater. In the dark, I found the silence and the magnificence of the desert to be peaceful. With no light pollution, the stars appeared endless, shone brighter and felt a lot closer to earth. I stood in solitude, no one around except the poisonous snakes and scorpions in search of food. Eventually, I had enough of bathing in the desert's tranquility and drove back to the Ranch.

The race started early the next morning with bearable heat at around 70 degrees Fahrenheit. One hundred eleven of us braved the elements and supported one another on the adventure. At the start of the race, I met an old friend who had moved to the desert the year before and ran the 135-mile Badwater Ultra. He told me that he had not been happy with his finish time and now trained to run it better this year. For this marathon, he aimed for a three hour and twenty-minute finish, which he missed by about ten minutes yet placed tenth among the finishers. The race director had a good sense of humor and reminded us that the white line on the side of the freeway (California Highway 190) would be our best friend for the day. We were advised to stay on the line to avoid both the oncoming cars and the creatures of the desert. I have been told that the Badwater Ultra runners stay on the cooler white line to avoid the scorching asphalt in the heat of the summer that could melt the outsoles of their shoes.

The course stayed below sea level and we were surrounded by desert wilderness and panoramic vistas of the mountains of Death Valley. As the temperature rose, a few slight hills on the course were enough to make breathing a challenge. The scenery became the same after a few miles and I focused on a few speeding oncoming cars. When they got close, I had no choice but to step into the desert, making sure not to trample any scorpions. The hills, the warming dry air and the head wind on the way out helped with the monotonous racecourse. We ran the same shoulder from Furnace Creek to Salt Creek and back. The beauty of the desert that I had experienced the day before soon became a distant memory. At times, it felt like I was on the treadmill running in one place looking at a picture of the desert.

Thank goodness I had my 16-ounce water bottle with me. Water stops were placed every three miles and I would drink almost all the water in my bottle by the time I hit the next aid station. The turn-around point was marked by a volunteer standing in the shade of an umbrella next to his car on the side of the road. He recorded our bib numbers while we turned and headed back to the finish. As the sun came over-head, the conditions grew intense. Somewhere on the way back, I saw a runner sitting on the side of the road suffering from heatstroke. I gave him all the water I had and ran back a mile to the last aid station asking for help. By the time I made it back to the same spot, someone had picked him up. The couple of extra miles that I added to the race, getting help for the runner in need, had taken its toll. Those runners left out there with me were not in good shape either. From mile 20 until the finish, the heat had risen to above 100-degree Fahrenheit, which slowed me down. A couple of miles before the finish another runner showed signs of dehydration, I gave him the water left in my bottle. By then, the race director was patrolling the course with plenty of water in his car. He filled my bottle and took the injured runner to the finish area.

In the last mile, the race director grew impatient with runners who would not take his offer for a ride to the finish. I saw him multiple times on the road stopping for the runners in trouble to give them a ride to the finish. I am sure a few took him up on his offer and earned a "DNF" (Did Not Finish), but others refused, which frustrated him. Half a mile before the finish line, a friend passed me while cussing at himself. He wondered why he was even out there. When I saw him at the finish, his arm was badly bruised, but not in a cast. He said that he had broken it a few weeks ago in another race (which explained the bruising) but he did not want to miss out on running a race in the desert. For those of us who race distances, we tend to have an appreciation for why someone would run a race with a broken arm. Although they have their own reasons, I have come to understand that participating in these challenges gives most of us a false sense of being immune to greater injuries, which can prove to be fatal.

After the finish, most of us did not want to hang around in the heat of the desert. We stayed for a little while, exchanged a few stories about the day, had snacks and rushed to get indoors. I had a flight out of Las Vegas that afternoon. I took a quick shower at the Ranch, checked out and drove through the desert to go home. Even though it was February, the grueling heat made me feel as though I had run the Badwater Ultramarathon after all. I cannot imagine how people could ever survive in Death Valley and I have a whole new respect for anyone who chooses to live in the desert.

As a funny side note, I learned a valuable geography lesson due to this marathon. Because I ran with the goal of completing a marathon in each state, I thought Death Valley would be the perfect opportunity to cross Nevada off my list, so I signed up for the race. Much to my surprise, I later learned that Death Valley is in Eastern California. Eventually I went back to Las Vegas, Nevada to run the Las Vegas Marathon. This did not bother me because these types of errors have introduced me to new places and experiences I never would have had otherwise.

Marathon Number 69
Death Valley Marathon
February 2012

Great Salt Desert : Dasht-e Kavir (Persian: دشت کویر, lit. ‹Low Plains› in classical Persian, from khwar (low), and dasht (plain, flatland), also known as Kavir-e Namak (lit. ‹salty lowlands›) and the Great Salt Desert, is a large desert lying in the middle of the Iranian Plateau. It is about 800-kilometre-long (500 mi) by 320-kilometre-wide (200 mi) with a total surface area of about 77,600 km2 (30,000 sq mi), making it the world's 24th largest desert.[1] The area of this desert stretches from the Alborz mountain range in the north-west to the Dasht-e Lut in the south-east. It is partitioned among the Iranian provinces of Khorasan, Semnan, Tehran, Isfahan and Yazd.
https://en.wikipedia.org/wiki/Dasht-e_Kavir

Death Valley - Death Valley is a desert valley in Eastern California, in the northern Mojave Desert, bordering the Great Basin Desert. It is one of the hottest places on Earth, along with deserts in the Middle East and the Sahara.
https://en.wikipedia.org/wiki/Death_Valley

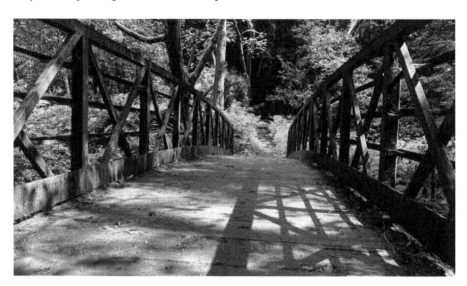

Running through the Amish country

For my Pennsylvania marathon race, I chose to participate in the Fifth Annual Garden Spot Village Marathon, which also offered a Marathon Relay and Half Marathon for others. Garden Spot Village is a retirement community for the disadvantaged and each year it benefits from this race. I picked the Lancaster County, Pennsylvania location because the area is home to both Amish and Mennonite families. I am always curious about the world we live in; travel expands my horizon.

The day before the race, after a red-eye flight into Philadelphia and driving a couple of hours west, I arrived in New Holland, Pennsylvania half asleep. A local lady working at the café next to the hotel warned me that the racecourse was challenging. At the small expo the day before the race, I waited for the pasta dinner to be held near the packet pick-up at the Garden Spot. They kept on postponing the dinner and, since I was not too hungry, I left the expo and drove around for a few hours. I stopped at a village with the unique name of "Intercourse". While there, I picked up a few souvenirs for my family and sampled some of the salsa made by Amish ladies at the tourist center before driving to Lancaster. At Lancaster, I saw nothing special, so I turned around and went back to New Holland.

A brisk spring morning heralded the start of the race, which kicked off on the 104-acre campus of Garden Spot Village adjacent to New

Holland in northeastern Lancaster County. The race began near the Legacy Garden, then traveled east for about two miles. The course circled around west for 12 miles through the Amish farmlands at the foot of Welsh Mountain before looping back to campus. Half- and full marathoners ran together for the first seven miles and then the 13.1-mile group turned back while the longer distance runners carried on. That marked the end of road closures and I was left to navigate cars and buggies until returning back to that split-off point.

Many unique experiences arose for me because of the location of this marathon. I ran through communities that live in a vastly different culture than is usually found in the United States. I even ran with some of the residents of these communities. Seeing young Amish men and women running the race was a unique experience. They ran in their traditional clothing, the men dressed in long dark pants, beige dress shirts and suspenders while the young women were covered in long sleeves, bonnets and long skirts. Both men and women wore shoes that did not resemble running shoes which made their running all the more impressive; they ran the hills as hard and strong as their horses did.

I thrilled at the scenery during this time of year. Farmers tilled the fields with horse-drawn plows and people traveled the roads in horse and buggies. Amish and Mennonite families watched the runners go by in a classic Lancaster County scene. They welcomed us as we ran through four of their townships. Watching the Amish kids looking at runners with wide eyes was an interesting sight.

The best sight for me was in the first mile of the race when I spied two neatly dressed Amish young boys as they sat on the porch of their farmhouse in the early morning hours just to watch us pass by. During the race, a few kids waved at us with the permission from their parents nearby, while many of them sat and played in the dirt as if we did not exist.

Running on roads with buggies all around (they are pulled along a lot faster than one thinks) was challenging, but I considered that a secondary obstacle. The primary obstacle was the organic "Lancaster road sod" courtesy of the horses. It lay everywhere on both the closed and open roads. Admittedly, the smell of freshly plowed fields with the horse and heavy wooed manure in the back overwhelmed me for the first few miles. As the wind picked up so did the dust of organic fertilizers, which made it difficult to breathe!

After the first few miles the road opened to traffic. As luck would have it, a horse auction was being held nearby and the roads were crowded mostly with horses and buggies. I found it quite picturesque when I ran toward them while they sat together with cars at the stop signs waiting for us to cross. Those types of amazing images have burned in my memory. In the later miles of the marathon, I found it scary to cross some of the major roads with no one to hold the traffic. Cars maneuvered too close to me as they tried to pass the horses and buggies. As mentioned earlier, horse droppings (also locally known as "road apples") added a whole different layer to the paved road, but the smell was strong enough to keep me awake.

The cheerful and supportive volunteers at the aid stations were the town residents of the Garden Spot Village. The weather warmed up later in the day; however, the wind and the hills were never ending. A runner who ran the race last year, claimed that there was only one hill in this course. After running it, I understood that the whole course was just one long hill!

After the race, I hung around and talked to the nice volunteers from Garden Spot Village and a few runners. Surprisingly, this small race had a great selection of post-race food for the participants. Along with plenty of water, they served Gatorade, chocolate milk, juice, coffee, tea, hot chocolate, soda, yogurt and amazing yogurt smoothies with whey protein powder. For food, they had ice cream, fruit wedges, trail mix, chips, pretzels, Rice Krispy treats and homemade oatmeal (with raisins and brown sugar). I had some oatmeal and fruit and then walked back to the hotel about half a mile away. I did not learn until later that they had also provided showers, hot tubs and a swimming pool at the finish!

The next day my plan had been to sleep in and leave late in the day for Philadelphia; however, looking out of the window around 5:00 a.m., I saw snow starting to fall and the weather report did not look good. I took a quick shower, had breakfast and left for the airport in the dark. About twenty minutes out of town, traffic came to a halt because of a jack-knifed truck. The freeway had closed. An hour later the police and fire department opened a single lane for us to pass. The nearly two-hour drive in the snow with no chains was scary, especially since I passed a few more accidents. Once I returned the car, I was relieved that the helpful agent at the airport got me on an earlier flight to my connection in Chicago. I did not want to get stuck in Pennsylvania if flights were canceled due to heavy snow. This was a spring storm primarily hitting the east coast, so I knew Chicago would have very little snow. After a few hours of waiting in Chicago due to multiple delays, I finally got on my flight home with fond memories of the run through Amish country fresh in my mind and nose.

Marathon Number 84
New Holland, PA
April 2013

The *Amish* (/ˈɑːmɪʃ/ - Pennsylvania German: Amisch; German: Amische) are a group of traditionalist Christian church fellowships with Swiss German and Alsatian Anabaptist origins. They are closely related to Mennonite churches.
https://en.wikipedia.org/wiki/Amish

Mennonite – Are members of certain Christian groups belonging to the church communities of Anabaptist denominations named after Menno Simons (1496–1561) of Friesland.
https://en.wikipedia.org/wiki/Mennonites#:~:text=The%20Mennonites%20are%20members%20of,1496%E2%80%931561)%20of%20Friesland

Intercourse, Pennsylvania – Is the heart of the Amish Country in Lancaster County. Intercourse (formerly known as "Cross Keys") is a business hub for both Amish and local folks. Beautiful Amish farms surround the village, which help make it one of the top tourist destinations for visitors to Pennsylvania Dutch Country.
https://lancasterpa.com/intercourse/

Welsh Mountain – Welsh Mountain Nature Preserve is one of Lancaster County's few remaining natural areas. An area of wooded slopes and rock outcroppings, this land supports a diversity of plant and animal life.
https://www.lancasterconservancy.org/preserves/welsh-mountain/

Buggies - A carriage pulled by a horse. In the United States and Canada, the word buggy typically refers to four-wheeled carriages, while in the U.K. and India it refers to two-wheeled ones. In parts of the U.S. and Canada, people such as the Amish use buggies for transportation.
https://www.dictionary.com/browse/buggy#:~:text=Most%20commonly%20it%20refers%20to,Amish%20use%20buggies%20for%20transportation

Jackknifing - Refers to the folding of an articulated vehicle so that it resembles the acute angle of a folding pocket-*knife*. If a vehicle towing a trailer skids, the trailer can push the towing vehicle from behind until it spins the vehicle around and faces backwards.
https://en.wikipedia.org/wiki/Jackknifing

Lost in Wilmington

The planning for this race seemed relatively easy, but I had not planned on my suffering from a painful herniated disk in my lower back. Two weeks before the race I believed that I would be able to shake it off. However, in a rush for a quick recovery, I aggravated it even more by getting a massage, attending my core class and having a friend help me with the wrong stretches.

After a long delay due to a fuel leak, I boarded the plane in San Francisco heading for Philadelphia. I took half of a prescribed pain killer so I could sleep during the red-eye flight. I awoke groggy only to realize we had been sitting on the runway for a couple of hours because of another mechanical problem. Finally, the captain reassured us as to the safety of the plane and we took off. The turbulence and my sore back woke me up quite a few times during the overnight flight. Once we landed and I dragged myself to a shuttle for the 45-minute ride to Wilmington, Delaware, I still did not know how I would be able to run the next day. I kept taking Aleve throughout the afternoon and managed to walk a mile and a half from the hotel to the expo where I was happy to see friends from the Fifty States Marathon Club.

I asked for advice from a seasoned runner at the club and he recommended taking it easy during the race and giving myself extra time by starting the race early. He advised me to ask the race director for an early start and for me to take two 500mg Tylenol every hour during the race. Medicating myself throughout the race seemed extreme and I decided to think about it. I did speak with the controlling director, who was busy taking care of every detail himself before the race debrief at the expo. He told me to be at the start around 5:45 a.m. to check-in for the 6:00 a.m. early start the next morning. The reunion of the Fifty States Marathon Club met outdoors by the expo. The folding chairs they had set up for us were very uncomfortable, so I stood for the club meeting but still felt the pain radiating though my lower back and down my leg. I excused myself and went back to the hotel, then spent the rest of the day in bed reading and turned in early.

The marathon began a couple of miles from my hotel. A shuttle from the hotel to the start was scheduled to depart at 5:05 a.m.. I stepped outside around 4:50 a.m. and took a deep breath; the fresh cold air perked me up. The streets were wet from a heavy rain during the night and I decided not to wait for the shuttle but took a brisk walk to the start, hoping it would help with my lower back pain. The passing police cars with sirens blaring made me think that maybe I had made a mistake to walk to the starting line through the rough downtown neighborhood. Too late to go back to the hotel for the shuttle, I continued walking and, in the dawn's light, I came across a few strange looking, yet harmless, characters.

After checking in with the race director, I met up with a couple of friends from the Fifty States Marathon Club who were also starting the race early. We were told that the racecourse was well marked, and we did not need a map to follow it. Our small group got sent off with one police bike escort and two volunteers on their bicycles leading us. We had been told not to pass the bikes since the first two miles of the racecourse had been changed. Apparently, the heavy rain overnight caused the Cape Fear River to burst its banks and flood part of the downtown area. Soon, I found myself passing up our small group and following one of the volunteer bikes that moved at a faster pace. As it turned out, that volunteer did not know the revised course and we became lost. Luckily, the police escort had followed us and guided us back to the right course. To do that, we looped back around by the start line where we were cheered by the roar of the puzzled runners lining up before the 7:00 a.m. race start. Their looks indicated that they were unaware of the early start and not sure what to make of the officer on a bike with me following him. From the reaction of the crowd, I figured the scene must have looked impressive. Distracted by being lost in the first mile of the race and inspired by the encouraging runners, I had forgotten all about my back pain!

After passing the start line, I moved fast to catch up with the police bike ahead of me. He led me to mile 2.5 and told me that now I would be on my own. I looked back at the course, saw no one and started to get concerned. They had marked the course with flour on the pavement the day before. Heavy rain during the night had washed away all of those markings. At mile three, I found the mile marker but no signs pointing which way to go. Being left-handed, I took a chance and went left. After a few hundred yards, orange cones appeared on the street but were they set up for the runners? A policeman, who sat in his patrol car to stay sheltered from the cold, saw my puzzled look and hesitation, rolled down his window and told me that I was on the right track there in the residential neighborhoods of Wilmington.

Early start meant that I had to make sure to look out for traffic lights in order to cross the street. The police patrol did not come out for the early start runners. They braved the cold only when the lead runner showed up so they could stop traffic for the regular start runners. One officer kindly got out of his car when I got close to one of the intersections and stopped the traffic so I could cross the street. Still with no runners behind me at mile marker five, I came upon the aid station, happy to see volunteers there. I asked them for directions, but no one knew the racecourse. They were busy setting up their aid station and getting ready for the crowd that would start the race at 7:00 a.m.. One of the volunteers told me to go across the bridge over the river ahead of me. I crossed the bridge and continued for a quarter of a mile only to find a turnaround sign. Not sure if it was related to the race, I ran back and saw two runners leaving the aid station. Assuming that they would go over the bridge and turn around as I did, I sped up over the hill opposite the bridge to keep ahead of them. I kept looking behind me but saw no one. I got worried that I might be lost again until I spied a sign with a number six by a parking garage and so continued on. Much to my relief, I saw a couple of race volunteers in orange vests at an intersection and stopped to ask them if I was on the right course. They told me they were merely traffic control and unfamiliar with the racecourse. I continued running in the hopes of seeing mile seven, but after half a mile I came across mile marker 26.

Because of my throbbing herniated disk, I had followed my friend's advice and taken two Tylenol before the start of the race. I blamed the medication for having confused the mile markers. When, once again, I found myself back at the start line, I decided I had gone the wrong way after the aid station at mile five. I asked another volunteer, who also did not know the course. I began to think this could all be thanks to the race director who wanted to control everything, as I had observed the day before at the expo. Witnessing my dilemma, a sympathetic spectator gave me a city map, useless at the time, but I thanked him for his kindness. Since I found myself at the start of the race, I believed it would be best to join the group of runners who had just begun their race. I thought if I followed them, I would not get lost again.

As for the actual marathon, the few hills on the course challenged me, especially running downhill with my lower back pain. My biggest fear revolved around my back freezing up to the point I could not even walk. But the race had its distractions. At mile 22, two of the volunteers argued vehemently, cussed at each other and were ready for a fistfight when I passed by. This counted as a whole new experience for me during a race. Also, before mile 24, a young lady sat on the curb next to an ambulance and had an oxygen mask on while her boyfriend made frantic phone calls. When I saw the uphill at mile 25, I decided to walk and not take a chance on further aggravating my back. I had taken two more Tylenol during the five-hour run. After crossing the finish line, I got my finisher's medal and some food. For me, the race had turned out to be 26.2 miles plus an extra seven miles of being lost. I still puzzled about that mile marker six I had seen before arriving at mile marker 26. After the race, I asked the director about that specific marker, he told me it could have been the sign for the daily parking fee of the garage, which was $6.00!

I looked for a cab or shuttle to return to my hotel only to find none available. I walked gingerly back to the hotel for a hot shower and rest before going to the airport. The wait at the airport and the six-hour flight home challenged my lower back pain. By the time I arrived, the pain was shooting down my left leg. The next day I visited my doctor's office to find out that I had an excruciating case of sciatica caused by the herniated disk in my lower back, the extra miles and the plane ride. For the next two months I followed my doctor's orders and rested, rehabilitated and restored my herniated disc and sciatica. Why? So I could get out there and run more marathons!

Marathon Number 86
Delaware Running Festival
Wilmington, DE
May 2013

Herniated disk - Is a condition that can occur anywhere along the spine, but most often occurs in the lower back. It is sometimes called a bulging, protruding, or ruptured disk. It is one of the most common causes of lower back pain, as well as leg pain or "sciatica."
https://orthoinfo.aaos.org/en/diseases–conditions/herniated-disk-in-the-lower-back/#:~:-text=A%20herniated%20disk%20is%20a,leg%20pain%20or%20%E2%80%9Csciati-ca.%E2%80%9D

Fifty States Marathon Club - The club is a non-profit organization dedicated to the promotion of health and fitness and the members share the common goal of running a marathon in each of the fifty states. To join, a runner must have completed a marathon in at least ten states.
http://www.50statesmarathonclub.com/#:~:text=The%20club%20is%20a%20non,in%20at%20least%20ten%20states

Sciatica - Refers to pain that radiates along the path of the sciatic nerve, which branches from your lower back through your hips and buttocks and down each leg. Typically, sciatica affects only one side of your body
https://www.mayoclinic.org/diseases-conditions/sciatica/symptoms-causes/syc-20377435#:~:text=Sciatica%20refers%20to%20pain%20that,one%20side%20of%20your%20body

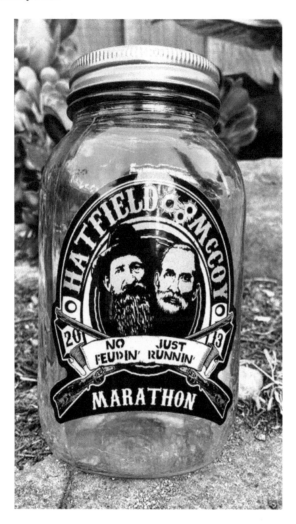

Hatfield-McCoy Feud

According to Wikipedia: The Hatfield–McCoy feud, also described by journalists as the Hatfield–McCoy war, involved two rural American families of the West Virginia - Kentucky area along the Tug Fork of the Big Sandy River the years 1863–1891. The Hatfield's of West Virginia were led by William Anderson "Devil Anse" Hatfield, while the McCoy's of Kentucky were under the leadership of Randolph "Ole Ran'l" McCoy. Those involved in the feud were descended from Joseph Hatfield and William McCoy (born c. 1750). The feud has entered the American folklore lexicon as a metonym for any bitterly feuding rival parties.

Having read the history between the two families, I was curious to visit the places the feud made famous. I also looked forward to running the setting where some of the most famous Kentucky/West Virginia events transpired. With plenty of hills and roads open to traffic, the racecourse offered plenty of physical and mental challenges to the runners. At the start of the race, the Marathon Maniacs Club had a strong presence. There were a handful of my running club members, the Fifty State Marathon Club, whom I met up with before the start of the race. The timing of the race coincided with the Hatfield and McCoy Festival and, as a result, a lot of activities took place in small towns surrounding Williamson in West Virginia.

I flew from San Francisco to Charleston, West Virginia for an over-night stay. Despite booking ahead of time, the car rental company at the airport in Charleston did not have the compact car that I had reserved, so they offered me a small pick-up truck. It was a basic truck with the older style radio antenna screwed on the front hood near the windshield. Once I picked up the vehicle, I noticed the screw was loose and tightened the antenna rod so that I would not lose it. After checking into the hotel late in the evening near the airport, I found a fast-food place nearby just before it closed. There were no customers when I walked inside. While waiting for my food two strange looking guys walked in, one sat across from me by the window and the other looked at me before walking outside. After a few minutes, I got suspicious and went outside to check on the pick-up truck in the poorly lit parking lot. To my surprise, the guy who had walked out was busy unscrewing the radio antenna. I casually walked up to him and asked him if I could help. I startled him and he ran away fast from the restaurant. The other guy, who watched us from the window, ran outside and took off on foot behind his friend. Standing in the parking lot, I could only smile. I walked up to the vehicle, unscrewed the antenna and threw it on the front seat before walking back inside to get my food. The next morning, I put the antenna back so that I could listen to the radio on my long drive to the race expo at Belfry High School in Kentucky.

With my navigation device acting up, I had to stop by a gas station to get directions to the race expo at the Belfry High School in Kentucky. When I arrived, the friendly volunteer high school students were more than accommodating in getting me soft drinks and napkins. Later I would learn that around 650 people in town volunteer at this race and a lot of businesses rely on the income generated from the race. The region had suffered from the shutdown of most of the coal mines nearby.

Since I had not been able to find a hotel near the start of the race, I planned to stay at a place in Matewan, West Virginia, a half an hour drive away from Belfry. The road to Matewan followed the same route as the first half of the marathon. With no signal on my GPS device, I was told by the volunteers at the High School to keep the Tug Fork River to my left as I drove toward Kentucky. The marathon would take place on the border between Kentucky and West Virginia with the first half of the race would be in Kentucky and the second half in West Virginia. The speed limit on the road to Matewan was 35-45 miles per hour; however, all the locals knew the roads well and drove over 50 miles per hour. On my drives back and forth from Matewan on that two-lane road, I pulled over a few times to let the local cars go by. I mostly passed through mining towns and saw cargo trains full of coal that stretched for miles.

Matewan is a town in Mingo County, West Virginia across the river form Pike County in Kentucky, at the confluence of the Tug Fork River and Mate Creek. The population was 499 in the 2010 census. When I entered this tiny mining town in the late afternoon, I saw kids dressed in Civil War gear holding Confederate flags and rifles and waving at me. Charles, the manager of the Coal Miners Cove where I would be staying, waited for me by the side of the road. This gave me some indication that his place did not host many visitors. Miners Cove had only four rooms situated next to a large open field. Walls and gates enclosed the field that opened on to the river dividing West Virginia and Kentucky. It appeared that the field had significant historic value. I could see lots of tents, cannons, displays of rifles and people dressed up as Civil War soldiers. I was exhausted from my journey and knew I had to get up early to drive back to Williamson for the start of the race. I tried to sleep but the sound of some funky 70's music next door made it difficult to close my eyes. I finally dozed off but woke up to the loud boom of a cannon that shook the building. The "soldiers" in the field were re-enacting a battle from the Civil War by firing cannons and shooting blanks from their rifles. This went on for at least half an hour. Tired from my long trip, I was not amused.

Starting out in the dark early the next morning, I took a different route to Williamson (HWY 49), which was more like a country road. Since my navigation device did not work due to a lack of satellite coverage, I could not be sure that I was headed in the right direction. What relief I felt when, after 45 minutes of driving, I finally saw some lights in the distance and it turned out to be the town of Williamson. This town would be the site of the race finish. The race guide indicated that all participants should park around the town of Williamson and catch shuttle buses to the start of the race at Food City (a grocery store) a mile down the road in South Williamson, Kentucky. This allowed us to have our transportation close to the finish line.

From the town of Williamson, they shuttled us to the start of the race in Food City's parking lot. In the dark, two race directors dressed as Hatfield and McCoy posed with the runners in the parking lot of the grocery store. The race started with the firing of a shotgun. We ran 13.1miles to Matewan which was the finish line of the half marathon. They celebrated the finishers by shooting off cannons and the ground under our feet shook.

We continued the race out of Matewan, through rolling hills on a muddy trail. We encountered a stranded half marathon runner who had followed her car's GPS after her race and gotten lost on the narrow muddy trail. We found it tricky to maneuver around her car. She drove her car up the hill ahead of us, figured she was going the wrong way, then came back and we had to scramble out of the way to avoid her as she drove toward us. Once we extricated ourselves from that experience, we went over a short swinging bridge and onto another highway that was open to cars and trucks. At around mile 23, as we were running up a steep hill facing the traffic, we had a scare when a large utility truck nearly hit the runner in front of me. I am not sure if it was intentional but, when the runner started cussing at the driver, I jumped off the road into a dry creek bed, but the truck still passed me too closely.

Most cars and trucks were courteous, and I found the volunteers on this race to be amazing, friendly and helpful. Two contradictory scenes I witnessed were a lady puffing on her electronic cigarette before the start of the race, and a young runner smoking a cigarette after the race.

At the finish, we were given finishers' medals and an empty Mason Jar with the logo of the race imprinted on the jar. This may have to do with the Kentucky moonshine. After the race, they served pulled-pork sandwiches and had other good tasting food and fruit. The weather warmed up by then and the humidity was high. I drove back to Matewan to find that they were taping a reality television show of the modern Hatfield and McCoy family and staging a tug-of-war over the river. Watching the fiasco, complete with cannons being shot, I marveled at how the reality television show's directors orchestrated their shoot. I went to an early dinner in town at a barbecue place and asked for a beer with my meal only to find out they did not serve alcohol. The server informed me that I could pick up a beer from the liquor store down the block and drink it in their restaurant. After I told her that I was too tired from the marathon to walk down the block, she brought me one of her own beers that a customer had given her earlier that day. I took her up on the offer and she quickly poured it into a disposable cup so that the contents could be disguised. She offered me a second, which I accepted. I left her a big tip when I left.

The next day, while I filled the car with gas out of Matewan, I noticed that at least a quarter of the store at the gas station was stocked with tobacco products. In fact, tobacco products have a great popularity in the region and occupied a large section of all the stores I visited. That being said, I found most places to be exceptionally clean and the people fairly friendly. From what I saw as I figured out my way around the town and during the marathon, I would like to go back to Matewan someday with my family so we might learn more about the history of the region.

Marathon Number 88
Hatfield McCoy Marathon
West Virginia / Kentucky
June 2013

Marathon Maniacs Club – This is a *club* for runners who are crazy about *running* marathons and are ready to take it to the next level.
https://www.marathonmaniacs.com/

50 States Marathon Club - The *club* is a non-profit organization dedicated to the promotion of health and fitness and the members share the common goal of running a *marathon* in each of the 50 states in the United States.
http://www.50statesmarathonclub.com/

Electronic Cigarette – A device that has the shape of a cigarette, cigar, or pen and does not contain tobacco. It uses a battery and contains a solution of nicotine, flavorings, and other chemicals, some of which may be harmful. When electronic cigarettes are used, the nicotine solution turns into a mist that can be inhaled into the lungs. The amount of nicotine in individual e-cigarettes can vary. It is not yet known whether electronic cigarettes are safe or if they can be used to help smokers quit smoking. Also called e-cigarette.
https://www.cancer.gov/publications/dictionaries/cancer-terms/def/electronic-cigarette

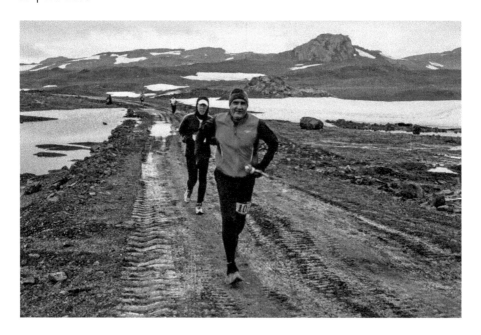

No Trace

When I boarded the Australian airliner in San Francisco for my connecting flight in New Zealand, the smiling attendant asked me if I were coming or going. His question took a few minutes to register due to his heavy "Aussie" accent. I responded I was going and took my seat for the long overnight flight. Packed like sardines in the economy class, I found it difficult to get any good shut-eye. Half asleep, I boarded my connecting flight to Santiago, Chile in Auckland, New Zealand. I hoped to get some sleep but, with heavy winds and turbulence on the smaller plane, I stayed awake and looked down on the earth below from 30,000 feet. A few seats ahead of me sat a couple that looked like runners. I wondered if they were "local" runners. When they had boarded the plane, I noticed the husband's T-shirt had San Jose imprinted on it, though I was not sure if it meant San Jose, California. They were friendly and courteous when we departed and went our separate ways. I got through customs in Santiago and, following the instructions from the race organizer, made it to the local terminal for my flight to Punta Arenas. Punta Arenas is a city near the tip of Chile's southernmost Patagonia region located on the Strait of Magellan that connects the Atlantic and Pacific Oceans. It is often used as a base for excursions to the surrounding Patagonian wilderness and Antarctica.

Our race schedule showed that we would run one marathon in Punta Arenas and another in King George Island in Antarctica; this way we would cover two continents in one trip.

It is always exciting to visit new places, get to know the people, and learn about their cultures, music and diet. Lack of sleep on the long flights made me drowsy as I walked through the gate to catch the flight on the last leg of my trip. A bus waited for us down the stairs through the gate and it was packed by the time I squeezed myself in. The race director had sent us our gear package prior to our travel and a light jacket with the logo of the race identified each runner who wore them on the bus. We casually nodded and greeted one another and waited for a long time in the crowded bus for our delayed plane. Eventually they sent us back to the terminal. While waiting, I met a few of the runners in our group from different parts of the world who had been on the same flight with me. The couple on the earlier flight were from Northern California and, when we got to know each other better, I learned that they lived about half an hour from me. Later I encountered another nice couple that lived only ten minutes away from me. The adventure bonded all of us so tightly that we formed "Team Numb" after our trip and we still get together at least once a year. I also met other runners who had their stories and tried to stand out with their unique reasons for making this trip. After an hour, they called us back to the bus again. We crowded on a second time and finally made it to our plane and off to Punta Arenas. Now that I had met new friends, especially from my local area, the flight seemed shorter while we chatted to get better acquainted.

Around 3:00 p.m. on Friday, January 24, 2014, we landed in Punta Arenas, Chile. I shared a cab with an African runner who lived in Dubai. She spoke non-stop all the way to the hotel and bragged about the races she had run. She was overly excited and nervous at the same time. All I wanted was to check-in, get to my room and get some much-needed sleep. I had injured my lower back a month earlier, which had left me paralyzed for three days, and was still recovering. I had not even been sure if I could make this trip. The long flights did not do my back any justice and I felt the pain as I took the elevator to the second floor of the hotel. I looked forward to taking a couple of Tylenols, immersing myself in a hot shower, stretching my lower back and getting sleep. But, when I opened the door to my room, I heard a scream, and a half naked lady ran into the bathroom. Tired as I was, for a moment I stood there thinking that I had to share the room. I knew I had booked a private room and did not want to have a roommate. The scream and the slamming of the bathroom door sent me right back downstairs to the hotel desk. The lady behind the counter casually told me that there was a mix-up and they had sent me to the wrong room. I was relieved.

The next morning, when I arrived at the hotel's restaurant "Diego del Almagro" for the buffet breakfast, I discovered that runners had already picked their clans and closed the seating at their tables. I shared a couple's table from New York who happened to be seasoned runners and very humble about their accomplishments. However, once I asked the question about their favorite races, they had no shortage of running stories. The race director and his crew had their own tables. They made it clear that they had no desire to mix in with the runners and gave the impression that they enjoyed a higher ranking than the rest of us. Later they reinforced this hierarchy by designating the first couple of rows on our transport buses for themselves. I find these behaviors to be fascinating case studies; my doctorate work is in management and one of the graduate courses I taught for over two decades is in organizational behavior.

We were told that we would be running the Punta Arenas marathon the next day; however, if the weather in Antarctica proved favorable, we would be on call to fly to King George Island instead for that marathon. Due to poor WIFI signals at the hotel, our mode of communication consisted of handwritten instructions from the race crew, posted by the elevators on the first floor.

After meeting a few more runners from different parts of the world, I ignored the notes posted by the elevators and headed back to my room for yoga and stretching my achy lower back. My main concern was how I would be able to run two marathons in a span of a few days, especially not being at all familiar with the course in Antarctica. In the early afternoon I decided to take a brisk walk around town and stretch my legs. In the hotel lobby, I was greeted by the race director and his crew who informed me that the forecast had cleared on King George Island, not to wonder too far from the hotel, check for instructions by the elevators and the tentative departure to Antarctica would be around 12:45 a.m. on Sunday. I stayed close by, found a place to exchange dollars to Chilean Pesos, visited a small local coffee shop in a basement a few blocks away from the hotel for a cup of tea and practiced my limited Spanish with the shopkeeper. On the way back to the hotel, I picked up a few greeting cards and stamps from a small shop; I intended to use them as souvenirs to be mailed from the post office in Antarctica.

Reading the handwritten instructions on colorful paper posted near the elevators, I learned that we were having a group dinner at 8:00 p.m. followed by the race director's briefing. We would be leaving for the airport at 10:45 p.m.. I packed for the race, followed by more yoga and stretching of my lower back before I went downstairs for the group dinner. I met a couple of runners from the Middle East who were obsessed with their running accomplishments in the Guinness Book of World Records and could not stop talking about them. Apparently, Guinness had a lot of customers in the Middle East and sold a lot of their books in that region. Later, I discovered that there were even more international runners in our group who proudly spoke of their running records. I did not mention that Antarctica would be my 97th marathon and ultra.

The briefing by the race director focused mostly on safety in Antarctica and instructions on evacuation if the weather changed for the worse. Also at the briefing, we were told of the zero-waste policy while on the island; all the waste had to come back with us to Chile. The race instructions were clear about carrying two filled water bottles and an extra urine bottle in case we needed it. The contents had to go back to Chile with us. Finally, the race director promoted his other adventures to the captive audience of 68 who would be running distances ranging from the half marathon to 50 kilometers on the white continent the next day. Outside the hotel, as we lined up to get into the buses for the airport, the air was filled with excited, nervous energy.

The small airport in Punta Arenas where we had landed the day before was deserted. The big electronic board in the lobby showed only one flight; DAP Airlines, Antarctica, 00:45. Most of us rushed to take pictures with the board while others made last minute adjustments to their gear and shoes. As I expected, once we boarded the flight, the race director and his crew sat in the front rows and the Chilean support crew occupied the rear seats. They would be stationed on the racecourse in immersion suit to make sure no one got lost and monitor that we did not leave any waste behind. After getting the clearance, we took off as scheduled for our two-hour bumpy flight on a specially equipped airplane to King George Island. Despite the turbulence, a full meal was served with choice of beverages during the flight, I am not sure how many of the passengers managed to eat. Surprisingly, an open bar was offered. I got a beer and saved it as a celebratory drink for after the race.

The cold air burned my lungs when we stepped off the plane in the dark and were immediately summoned to walk to the start line. The race crew kept busy unloading the supplies, then they took off ahead of us to set up a race tent and two teepee porta-potty tents at the start line. Once we dropped off our gear in the tent, runners rushed to form a line by the porta-potties. They came equipped with a bucket in the center of the tent and a 55-gallon drum. The instructions were to dump the bucket into the drum and clean up for the next person in line. The drums then would be sealed after the race and go back with us to Chile. We were not to leave any trace of us behind.

The race started at 3:19 a.m. in the dark with a temperature of zero degrees centigrade (low 30's Fahrenheit). Factor in the wind chill and the temperature that ended up being negative 8 degrees centigrade. The course consisted of running six laps of a 4.35-mile round-trip loop with a total elevation gain of 2,228 feet. When we reached the turnaround point, a couple of race crew occupying an old heavy-equipment cabin recorded our numbers while trying not to freeze in the cold. The sun came up after the first loop but the temperature with the wind chill dropped further. It was nice to see other runners with different paces as we passed each other on the repeated out-and-back.

Once by the tent at the start and finish area, we had access to our backpacks so that we could change gear according to the changing weather. The summer "heat" of Antarctica had melted the snow into ice on some parts of the course. There were also patches of deep gravel and frozen river rocks before the turn-around that caused a few injuries. Most of the course was covered in snow and the view of white hills and the ocean were a scene out of a well-cropped postcard. A few curious seals and penguins ventured out of the water and approached us throughout the course to find out what the commotion was all about. Being spared the damages caused by humans, they did not consider us a threat and provided many photo opportunities. The eight-hour cut-off was changed to seven after the race started because of the changing weather. This proved generous enough so we could take our time, enjoy the view, cheer each other on and pose for selfies.

With my pace slowing down and the wind chill temperature of negative18 degrees centigrade, it was difficult to think of another marathon in Punta Arenas upon our return to Chile. Halfway through the race, most of us were adding layers and began to show stronger support for each other on the course. Challenging experiences lead to stronger bonds and form lasting friendships. As mentioned earlier, "Team Numb" was born as result of this experience and, many years later, we are still in touch and continue to support one another.

Once I finished the race, I totally felt the cold and the Chilean's research camp kindly offered their small space to us so we could stay warm while others finished their races. A few people ventured out back on the course to take more pictures with the penguins, while others went to the small post office with the race crew to stamp our postcards. We enjoyed the company of the scientists at the camp who barely spoke English; one of them eagerly shared his research photos with me in exchange for my celebratory beer. We were lucky the weather mostly cooperated; everyone finished their race. As we walked back to the plane, I took a few minutes to reflect on the experience and enjoy the serenity of King George Island. Before boarding, I felt a tap on my shoulder and was surprised to see the Chilean base camp's scientist who had run to find me. While catching his breath and in his broken

English, he thanked me again for the can of beer and gave me a patch from his research camp as a souvenir. A can of beer must have been a precious commodity in the Southern Hampshire.

We exchanged stories on the flight back to Punta Arenas and could not stop talking about the porta-potty teepees for a few days after the race. A couple of days later, we ran our marathon in Punta Arenas before returning home.

Marathon Number 97
Antarctica Marathon
King George Island
January 2014

Aussie - The short form for an Australian, is pronounced for fun with a hissing sound at the end, it sounds as though the word being pronounced has the spelling Oz. Hence Australia in informal language is referred to as Oz.
https://timesofindia.indiatimes.com/Why-is-Australia-called-Oz/articleshow/2116820.
cms#:~:text=When%20Aus%20or%20Aussie%2C%20the,is%20referred%20to%20as%20Oz

Patagonia - Spanish pronunciation: [pataˈɣonja], is a sparsely populated region at the southern end of South America, governed by Argentina and Chile. The region comprises the southern section of the Andes Mountains, lakes, fjords, and glaciers in the west and deserts, tablelands and steppes to the east.
https://en.wikipedia.org/wiki/Patagonia#:~:text=Patagonia%20(Spanish%20pronuncia-tion%3A%20%5Bpata%CB%88%C9%A3onja,and%20steppes%20to%20the%20east

Immersion Suit - Also known as a survival suit or gumby suit, an immersion suit is an essential piece of survival equipment if you ever find yourself in a cold-water survival situation. Usually made from neoprene, survival suits are a special type of dry suit intended for emergency situations and designed for fast and easy donning.
https://www.survivalatsea.com/survival-suits.aspx#:~:text=Also%20known%20as%20a%20survival,for%20fast%20and%20easy%20donning

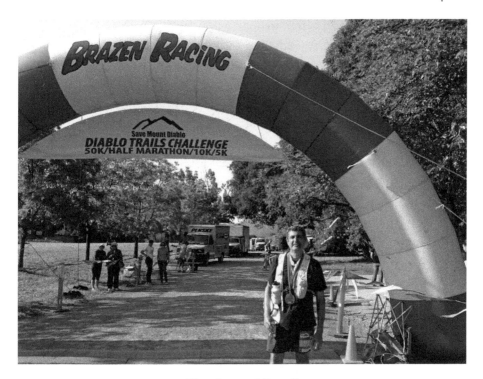

The Sacred Land

For me, trail running has become my preferred type of race. One magical place to find a variety of excellent trails is in Mount Diablo State Park and the preserved lands surrounding it. Mount Diablo stands out as a 3,849-foot-high solitary peak located 50 miles east of San Francisco and visible from most of the San Francisco Bay Area.

The park stretches for about 20,000 acres. Native Americans who once lived on the land and worshiped the mountain considered it to be sacred. According to Miwok and Ohlone mythology, Mt. Diablo was thought to be the point of all creation. Of the many trails on the mountain, the Trail Through Time, a 6.3-mile trek through 190 million years of geologic history, provides visitors a glimpse of this sacred land. Some of the giant rocks on the trail cradle the indentations where indigenous people used to grind acorns.

For my first race on Mt. Diablo, I chose the 50-kilometer distance so I could cover more of the trails on the mountain. The racecourse included public and private land. The private ones had offered a right-of-way through their property for the race. Not knowing the racecourse worked to my advantage since I was not familiar with the elevation gain of a combined 10,584 feet or the challenges associated with those climbs. Instead, I had merely set myself smaller goals of meeting the cut-off times at specific aid stations. However, I worried whether I could even accomplish that because I had been experiencing pain on both knees for the past few months. In addition, for six weeks prior to the race, I had been on a plant-based diet. The night before the race, I added meat to my dinner for extra protein. I struggled to get up at 3:00 a.m. on race morning due to a stomachache. Around 5:00 a.m. I forced down a bagel, hoping to clear my system before the race and the trick worked, at least psychologically. I drove to the town of Clayton, parked near the finish line in the dark with a few other cars and waited in the cold and windy dawn to catch the shuttle to the start at Castle Rock Park in Walnut Creek. Once in the shuttle, we got a quick briefing both on "Save Mt. Diablo" (a program to preserve, protect and restore its remaining 70,000 acres and foothills for wildlife and people to enjoy), and the race itself. The lady who spoke was a shy and nervous elite runner who turned out to be the female race record holder. Once we arrived at the parking lot at Castle Rock, we could not check-in for the race because our race bibs were in the last shuttle to arrive. After 40 minutes of waiting, we cheered when the last small bus pulled in. They had our bibs but no safety pins to secure them to our race shirts. Fortunately, I had put a few pins in my sweat bag the day before.

Before the race, a friend told me about a recent 50-mile event he participated in and how he did not make the cut-off at mile 48 and got pulled out of the race. He blamed it on a skunk in the early part of the course; he had spent over half an hour throwing rocks and branches at it to clear the trail so he could pass. His story motivated me to focus more on the cut-off times for the race so I would not miss them. With the delays, we started 20 minutes late and the race director announced that the cut-off times had changed as a result.

We began at an incline before running into meadows where cows darted away from runners while calling out in distress. A few tried to cross our path and we had to make sure not to step on their fresh cow patties. Out of the meadows came the first hill with no crest in sight. One of the runners, who had competed in the race before, told us that we had another 1.7 miles to go to reach the top. I could hear a few fellow runners grunting as we continued to climb. The course passed through some private properties on the mountain. There were a few farm gates that seemed to become human proof as the miles accumulated. Each had their own distinct mechanism and I would not be surprised if fellow runners climbed some of them instead of bothering with the latches. One of my friends caught up with me after the last gate and we ran on the windy ridge up to the first aid station together. The aid station was well stocked and the volunteers turned out to be experienced trail runners, which made them very accommodating to our needs and questions. The county's Search and Rescue Team was present and in full uniform. We had to check in with them to make sure that we had made the cut-off time.

In the briefing before the race we were told that, although the course was well marked, we were not supposed to get lost. If we did, Search and Rescue would be after us with our emergency contact person's phones ringing off the hook. We were left with no doubt that cut-off times would be strictly enforced. After each aid station, steep hills loomed and a few times I had to stop and catch my breath walking up them. I did not mind at all because the views were breathtaking, with a 360-degree panorama of the Bay Area over the windy ridges. A few riders on horses passed by me on the trails; they gently pulled their steeds to the side and offered words of encouragement. At the second aid station, I talked to a volunteer who told me about the upcoming narrow single-track trails with poison oak on both sides. Once I got to that section of the trail, I had no choice but to be brushed by the weeds and the poison oak. I passed a few runners who struggled on the steep climb and I was not sure if they made the last cut-off.

The endless hills were covered with tall grasses and tiny beautiful blue, orange and red wildflowers. I found it difficult to take in the views due to the fact I could not ignore the challenging steep down-hills followed by yet another uphill. Once, I passed by a coyote near the trail and warned the runner behind me to be vigilant going up the steep hill. That is when I realized we were traversing through wildlife territory. Lizards ran away from me and a few small snakes slithered on the trails. All the while, I made sure not to step on both fresh and old horse and coyote droppings.

My solo run to the aid station at mile 23 (37 kilometers) turned out to be one the most scenic parts of the course. An eerie feeling hung in the air and I made noises so that the wildlife would be aware of my presence. When I Arrived at the aid station on the mountainside where it was hotter, I was greeted by the Search and Rescue. I checked in, filled up my water bottles and my bandanna was removed by one of the volunteers. She soaked it in ice-cold water and it felt good to wrap it back around my neck. She asked if I wanted ice-chilled water poured over my head. Given the heat at the time, I nodded yes. I put my head forward to get my shower and gasped as the cold water dripped down my back. I heard a chuckle from one of the volunteers. I thanked her and told her I would be chilled for the next eight miles. Half a mile later, I realized that some of the water had gotten in my watch, but luckily it still functioned well.

The steep downhill toward the finish took a toll on both my injured knees and, for the first time in a race, I took an Aleve to ease the pain. Later, I learned my lesson about taking Aleve during races because, one day after another race, it eventually sent me to the emergency room with a kidney stone. That agonizing experience taught me not to take any more painkillers during races. Once I left the last aid station at around mile 28 (45 kilometers), one of the race organizers told me he would see me at the finish to take my photo. I knew then the end was in sight and picked up my pace while taking in the beauty of the trail.

I had enjoyed being out there, meeting new friends and taking the time to thank the volunteers at the aid stations. A mile before the finish, I startled a deer grazing next to the trail and watched it run ahead of me. I could not have asked for a better pacer as I chased the deer before it disappeared into the woods. Entering Castle Rock Park near the finish, a sign warned about the presence of wildlife. Besides coyote and deer, bobcats also lived in the park. Having encountered a bobcat on a trail before, I found them to be territorial and aggressive. I was relieved I had not encountered any on that day. The runners who had finished ahead of me cheered me on as I crossed the finish line. We all enjoyed our post-race meal together.

After running my first 50-kilometer race on the beautiful and challenging trails of Mount Diablo, I have returned often throughout the years to run and explore many of its other trails with friends in different seasons. In springtime, water flows in the creeks and wildflowers blanketing the sides of the mountain have stopped me in my tracks many times. Once, the summer heat caused me to suffer heatstroke near the peak and the experience humbled me. The high winds of autumn skirting the top of the open ridges near the peak have lifted me up off my feet for a better view of the surroundings. Winter brings fog, which has given me the feeling of running above the clouds in the higher elevations and, on rare occasions, snow falls but does not sit on the ground for too long. Running through many of the trails on the mountain has taught me respect for the natural beauty it has to offer. I have come to appreciate why this paradise became the sacred land of the indigenous people. I would encourage anyone to explore this phenomenal place.

Marathon and Ultra Number 101
Diablo Trails Challenge 50K
April 2014

Mt. Diablo - Is a mountain of the Diablo Range, in Contra Costa County of the eastern San Francisco Bay Area in Northern California. It is south of Clayton and northeast of Danville. It is an isolated upthrust peak of 3,849 feet (1,173 meters), visible from most of the San Francisco Bay Area. Mount Diablo appears from many angles to be a double pyramid and has many subsidiary peaks, the largest and closest of which is the other half of the double pyramid, North Peak, nearly as high in elevation at 3,557 feet (1,084 m) and is about one mile (1.6 kilometers) northeast of the main summit.
https://en.wikipedia.org/wiki/Mount_Diablo

Miwok Mythology – According to Miwok mythology, the people believed in animal and human spirits, and spoke of animal spirits as their ancestors. Coyote in many tales figures as their ancestor, creator god, and a trickster god. The Miwok mythology is similar to other Native American myths of Northern California.
https://en.wikipedia.org/wiki/Miwok_mythology#First_People

Ohlone Mythology - The mythology of the Ohlone (Costanoan) Native American people of Northern California include creation myths as well as other ancient narratives that contain elements of their spiritual and philosophical belief systems, and their conception of the world order. Their myths describe supernatural anthropomorphic beings with the names of regional birds and animals, notably the eagle, the Coyote who is humanity›s ancestor and a trickster spirit, and a hummingbird.
https://en.wikipedia.org/wiki/Ohlone_mythology

Search and Rescue – (SAR) is the search for and provision of aid to people who are in distress or imminent danger. The general field of search and rescue includes many specialty sub-fields, typically determined by the type of terrain the search is conducted over.
https://en.wikipedia.org/wiki/Search_and_rescue_in_the_United_States

Bay Area - The Bay Area (more fully, the San Francisco Bay Area), ringing the San Francisco Bay in northern California, is a geographically diverse and extensive metropolitan region that is home to over 7 million inhabitants in cities such as San Francisco, Oakland, and San Jose.
https://wikitravel.org/en/Bay_Area_(California)#:~:text=The%20Bay%20Area%20(more%20fully,%2C%20Oakland%2C%20and%20San%20Jose.

Aleve - A nonsteroidal anti-inflammatory drug (trademarks Aleve and Anaprox and Aflaxen) that fights pain and inflammation. synonyms: Aflaxen, Anaprox, naproxen sodium.
https://www.vocabulary.com/dictionary/Aleve#:~:text=Definitions%20of%20Aleve,%3A%20Aflaxen%2C%20Anaprox%2C%20naproxen%20sodium

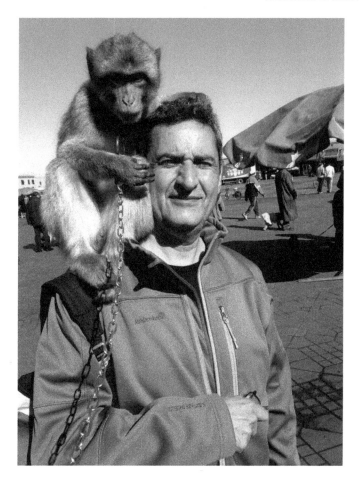

Memories of Marrakech

I arrived in Marrakech, Morocco just after dawn in January 2015, very much looking forward to completing my goal of a marathon on every continent. The race was scheduled for Sunday, the 25th of January and I looked forward to seeing more of this city on foot. Choosing Marrakech, Morocco as my last continent for a marathon had worked best with my schedule. The fear of an Ebola outbreak in sub-Saharan Africa a few months before the race made the decision easier. In addition, a running friend had told me that I would enjoy the race in this town. The trip had been generously arranged for me by a travel agent friend, who thought I should be immersed in the heart of the Moroccan culture. For him, that meant a week in the old city of Marrakech, by myself. I found the journey to be both a blessing and a curse.

Going through the passport control was smooth with no customs. Before the trip, I had read a little on the Internet about the culture and the notion of bargaining but was not prepared when I approached the taxi line outside of the airport. Soon seven to eight drivers offer a good deal surrounded me. Once I walked away from the 200 Dirham fare, or about US$50.00, I got offered a private SUV parked across the gate from where I came out of the airport for just 150 Dirham (about $40.00). Compared to the cars nearby and the neat way the driver was dressed, I became suspicious and declined that offer. In my research, I had also read about the emerging presence of ISIS in Morocco and the rise in kidnappings for ransom by them. I returned to the taxi driver who had approached me first, offered 150 Dirham and drove off with him. My lodging was at Dar Sohane in the old city, also known as the Medina.

Before dropping me off at the entrance to a bazaar, the driver drew me a map on a scrap of paper showing me where to go and how to maneuver my way through the bazaar. Later I found out there was an easier way to get to the hotel if only the taxi would have gone around to the town square called Jemaa el-Fnaa. Pulling my roller bag behind, I had to walk 150 meters or about 500 feet through the bazaar to my reserved hotel. I was greeted by strange looks from the shopkeepers and their customers. I said to myself that I was probably a curiosity to them because my Middle Eastern features made me seem as though I were Moroccan, but my American-style clothing identified me as a tourist. As I walked through the bazaar, there were occasional uninvited people who followed me, while the shopkeepers were inviting me to visit their stores and buy souvenirs. Traveling alone, jet-lagged and not knowing the culture, paranoia set in pretty quickly.

Walking the narrow path in the middle of the bazaar through a maze of shops, motorbikes, shoppers and curious looks, I took a right turn after the main mosque as instructed by the map on the scrap of paper. Halfway down an alley, a well-dressed young man with a big smile offered his help in English. For some reason I accepted his help and, after giving him the name of the hotel, I followed him. Soon another guy with dark glasses joined us from behind on the other side of the alley. As we entered a narrow alleyway, the walls grew and seemed to reach the sky, making the daylight disappear. I found myself between these two guys when they started to converse in Arabic. Being sleep deprived from the long flights, bargaining for a ride to the hotel, putting up with the stares in the bazaar, coupled with these so-called helpers speaking a different language, made me a little more paranoid, but I tried to keep my cool.

Just then I flash-backed to an experience last September in Bucharest, Romania, where my brother lives. My nephew and I went for an early morning walk; he wanted to show me how a driveway had been built that was completely blocked by an existing tree. He was interested in taking a picture for his social media post. We ended up on a quiet street with no one but a big Gypsy guy on his cell phone standing near a large black SUV in the middle of the street. As we passed by, he called out in Romanian. We ignored him and just kept walking. In the next block we were caught off guard when the same black SUV with three big guys came toward us on the wrong side of the street. My nephew claimed to be an expert in the Romanian culture, so he suggested we turn around and keep our slow pace without panicking. Soon three big guys were walking behind us, so close we could hear their breathing. We did not see a single car or person in the whole neighborhood. Occasionally, someone would look at us from their windows and then hide behind their curtains. We stayed calm and kept on walking until we no longer heard their footsteps. I was relieved when we turned onto another street, crossing over to the far sidewalk. However, just then, we were nearly run over by the same SUV with all those guys shouting at us. A time like this is when the fight or flight response kicks in. We chose the flight without a second thought. Running effortlessly in our street shoes, we both set new personal records for the next kilometer until we blended in with a crowd on a busy street near an outdoor vegetable market. We found our way to my brother's house and, once the gate was closed, I felt cold sweat running down my neck. I smiled and told my nephew that he should take up running.

Now, walking toward the hotel in the Medina of Marrakesh with one guy in front and being followed by another, I thought "how could there be a hotel in this neighborhood and why did I accept help and followed a stranger into these narrow dark alleys just because he smiled and spoke English?" The next turn took us into another quiet alley with nothing but a few closed doors. The voice of my martial arts trainer called to me "one block, one punch". My natural instincts kicked in and, in one automatic moment, I let go of my bag and executed those words into action. Next thing I knew I had the first young guy against the wall, my left hand squeezed hard on his throat and his eyes were popping out. Time slowed down to where I could not make out his screams and gasps for air. I only watched his lips moving and his face turning blue, then silence. A couple of pairs of eyes peaked from behind a door into the alley. I finally awoke from my dreamlike state and let go of his throat. After a few coughs, he mumbled with a broken voice, "I no lie to you, here…around the corner." Then I heard the sound of footsteps as both of them ran down the alley in the opposite direction.

Bag in hand and no one in sight in the quiet alley, I looked up searching for any written sign on the walls that could help me navigate my way out. I finally turned down another alley and found myself standing in front of an enormous double-sided wooden door with a small dead tree in a large cement vase next to it. A faded sign revealed the name of the hotel, "Dar Sohane". With adrenalin still pumping through me, I was breathing hard and a cold sweat was running down my neck as I banged rapidly with my knuckles on the wooden door. The door cracked open and the smiling face of Hamza greeted me by my last name. I let go a sigh of relief when he said they were expecting me. I walked behind him through a long dark tunnel toward the light of an interior courtyard. To my surprise, I found a graceful fountain containing a small pool of water where an abundance of red rose petals floated. Marble floors surrounded the fountain and charming tables and chairs were set up all around the courtyard. I saw a kitchen on my left and, to my right, a long room decorated with stunning Moroccan furnishings in colors of red and turquoise. Looking up, I could see three floors with three to four rooms on each floor. For a moment, I imagined myself in an old black and white movie with only me in it.

I asked Hamza if they had Wi-Fi, then sat at a small table near the water fountain in the center of the courtyard and connected to Viber. With the recent alley experience in the back of my mind, but not wanting to worry my wife, I sent her a message that I had made it and I would be checking in with her every 30 minutes for the next few hours. Hamza had disappeared into the kitchen; the place was disarmingly quiet. It was then I realized I was the only guest at a hotel located in some random alley somewhere in Marrakech. Having an Internet connection gave me some sense of security until I walked into the marble covered kitchen to find Hamza standing in front of me with a big knife in his hand. For a moment I froze as I gazed at the knife. He broke the silence, saying he was chopping mint to make me Moroccan tea and that he would be out in a few minutes.

Hamza showed up with a pot of tasty Moroccan mint tea and a plate of cookies. He then excused himself and quickly disappeared down the dark tunnel leading to the front door. I heard him open and shut the door and the key turn as he locked it behind him. This seemed oddly curious to me, so I got up to check on the door. My paranoia ramped up when I realized I could not open the door as it was locked from outside! Resigned, I walked back to the table, looked at the cookies and tea, looked up to the floors surrounding the courtyard and found only emptiness. I called out a few times, but no one responded; this is when I knew I was by myself. I took the stairs to the second floor only to find all the doors open and the elegantly decorated rooms empty. Same for the third floor. I even went to the rooftop to find an exit route; the only door I found was locked. There was no way out of this place. I tried to stay calm, but I felt a little dizzy. I sat on the edge of the steps looking down at the courtyard and the fountain. The now sinister-looking rose petals seemed like blood from this high up. I felt the side effects of a concussion from a running incident three years ago – dizzy and disoriented. Sleep deprived and staring at the rose petals in the water, I questioned myself about this running business and having goals such as running a marathon on each continent. With Africa being my last continent, would I survive the journey? Would I even make it safely to the start of this race? A surge of self-doubt added to my newly found paranoia. After a while, I went down and sent another message to my wife telling her all was good. I regarded the tea and cookies anew, wondering if they were tainted and if Hamza went out to bring extra help so that he could kidnap me.

I became more concerned when, looking around for my bag, I remembered Hamza had helped me with it when I entered and I had not seen it since. I turned and looked into the kitchen, assuring myself the knives were within reach should I need them. I poured myself a cup of mint tea, took a bite out of a cookie and told myself, "This is how it ends, somewhere in Marrakech in a hotel as the only guest and never completing my goal of runs on every continent."

I do not remember how much time passed before I heard the key turn in the lock. I jumped up and moved toward the kitchen. I have been in danger before, once when completing one of my 50 states' marathons. Someone had followed me for a block, in the dark, the night before the race. I ran fast toward the safety of the hotel lobby where I stayed, and the mugger could not keep up. This time felt different, I was trapped inside my hotel and very vulnerable. I found the biggest knife in the kitchen. The voice in my head said, "be present," it also reminded me to "win the war before it starts" (a quote from the Art of War). With the knife in hand, I stepped back into the courtyard, took a deep breath to slow down the time, sipped that strong mint tea infused with pounds of sugar and reminded myself that, with calm, the battle is won. The door opened. I felt a cold breeze come through the tunnel, followed by Hamza. There was no one with him; he stood there, looking at me holding the cup of tea in one hand, the knife in the other. Hamza, too, held a shiny metal object in his hand and asked me if I wanted more tea. I put down my teacup, walked calmly toward him and stared into his frozen eyes while standing inches away from him. For the second time that day I had entered the deep subconscious level of survival. Then I heard the sound of a metal object hitting the marble floor, saw Hamza jump back with his mouth open but no sound to be heard. We both looked at the floor. "That could not be a showerhead with a small pipe attached, could it?" I asked myself. As if I perceived him underwater, Hamza looked at me with his lips moving, but still no sound. In my heightened state, a few minutes felt like a few hours passed before I reached down, grabbed the showerhead and tried to hand it to him. He just stood there regarding me. Eventually, Hamza unfroze and, with trembling hands, took the showerhead. In his limited English, he told me that the previous guest had broken the shower head in my bathroom. He had simply gone out to get a new one. While walking up the steps toward my room, he said he would be down soon to make more mint tea and asked if I wanted more cookies. He also informed me that he had taken my bag to my room on the second floor earlier and had failed to mention it. I came back to reality, found myself holding the knife and staring at the rose petals in the water fountain. I no longer considered their blood-red color a threat. I sighed in relief, put the knife back in the kitchen and sat down. Hamza never mentioned the incident, as if it never happened.

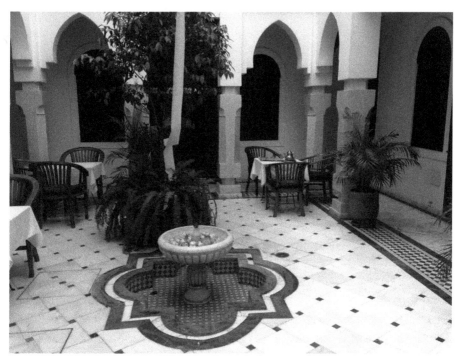

Hamza brought me a map of the old city and told me that the showerhead had been fixed so my room was ready. I went up to the second floor with a pounding head and tired legs. I soon learned that, as is customary in Moroccan architecture, the entrance to most rooms has a low circular arch before the actual door to the room. I was so busy admiring the colorful door that I missed seeing the archway and banged into it with my forehead. "What more could happen today?" I thought as I stumbled dizzily into the room and locked the door behind me. I turned around to find a beautifully appointed room with a marble bathroom fit for a king. I sent another message to my wife; by now she was concerned as to why I was checking in so often. I told her I missed her and our boys. She reminded me that she just dropped me off at the San Francisco airport yesterday. To me, I felt a world away and stuck in some African twilight zone while I fell into a deep sleep in the middle of the day. I woke up later in the afternoon and went down-stairs with the map in hand, now very wary of door arches. Hamza was on his computer in the lobby of the courtyard. A few candles burned on the tables by the water fountain. He offered tea. I thanked him and told him I had overdosed on the mint tea for the day. We both chuck-led as Hamza handed me a key to the front door.

Through the dark tunnel and out the door into the unforgotten alley, I went to navigate my way out of the maze of alleys and into the bazaar. Looking up, I noticed the signs on the tall alley walls pointing to Dar Sohane. This made me feel comfortable as I wended my way toward the town square. Before entering the bazaar, I saw the young man I had pinned against the wall earlier in the day. He paled when he saw me, took a step back and regarded me with uncertainty. This had not been a dream after all; my guilt set in as he froze. I walked up to him, reached out for a handshake. He reciprocated but his hand felt cold as he looked into my eyes. I said hello in Arabic. Only then did a faint smile appear. He muttered that I should come for a cup of tea at his father's shop and look at the carpets. He called his father "Hajji" – this is a title earned by those devoted Muslims who have completed the pilgrimage to Mecca. There is a belief that the practicing Muslims who have completed this pilgrimage, have secured themselves a place in heaven upon their passing. Handshake done, the cold of his hand imprinted in my mind, I thanked him in Arabic and promised to visit the next day. I could not predict what would await me in the shop, considering what had transpired today. Either way, I thought, the visit was going to cost me. Maybe the purchase of a small rug would mend the bridges.

"Only a small rug," said the voice in my head as I looked at the piles of colorful rugs in front of me the next day, all while holding a cup of Moroccan mint tea. Hours passed as Hajji went through the piles of rugs in the hope of selling his most expensive one, assuring me that he would be taking care of the transportation costs to the U.S. After all, his place in heaven is secured, so he was not worried if the tourist paid triple the price for that same rug. When I refused more tea, he got frustrated and left. His son took over and I finally picked out a small blood-red rug. Once we finished haggling over the price, I walked out with the rug under my arm feeling good that I paid half of the asking price. Actually, I would have not minded if I paid the full price for pinning an innocent man against a wall. "What I am going to do with a rug?" I asked myself when I walked into the bazaar. I thought that Hajji had taught his son well by having him learn multiple languages in order to give directions to the lost tourist as a way of luring them into their carpet shop.

Holding the map, I backtracked my way through the alley toward Dar Sohane. I saw kids playing soccer with a worn-out ball, covered in dust, yelling, fighting, laughing and acting like their favorite soccer player on television. I knew this because, in my youth, I was one of them. We played for hours in the alleys behind our house in Shahrud, Iran during the summer breaks. I walked in the middle of the alley through their game as if I were a shadow on the ground. They were so intent on playing in their own soccer universe that I am not sure if they could even see me. For once, I felt invisible and glad for the lack of usual curious stares I got from the rest of the locals. This was a special moment in my trip when I became one with those kids.

Soon I was back in the hotel for more mint tea and conversation with Hamza until more guests showed up and stayed for a day or two during their travels around Europe and Africa. Passing by the carpet shop in the next few days, I was greeted by a big smile from Hajji and we struggled for conversation. Each time I saw him, I was reminded of what I had done to his son and the voice in my head called out, "What would a jail look like in this city?" Instead, the interaction consisted of a deep breath, a gentle bow and a handshake, followed by As-Salaam-Alaikum (hello) and a ma'aasalaama (goodbye). A few meters later, I thought, "I should have asked for his son's name. What if we had the same name?"

Morocco is a land of contrast where religion fills the gap of illiteracy and, unlike India that can shock all senses at once, it manages to shock some of them most of the time. On a visceral level, the sounds, colors and flavors of Marrakech are organic and authentic. Both men and women have mixed African and European features stunning enough to make them ideal muses for the artist. If only I had a canvas and paint, I might have sat across from the beggars on the sidewalks of the bazaar and captured a few of them. The old town was alive at all hours, especially at night when the music was the loudest and the tourists were out. In the crowded Jemaa el-Fenaa, there were entertainers, snake charmers and performing monkeys. Shopkeepers left their doors open as they ran to the nearby mosque when the call to prayer sounded in the old city. They rushed back to their shops after prayers for mint tea or a meal. Their smiles showed off their worn-out, tobacco-stained teeth. Beggars lined up in the alley by the main mosque during the prayers. It appeared to be a custom of the worshippers to give money to the beggars so that the worshippers could wash out more of their sins, even after purification with prayers.

One beggar family caught my attention, and the memory has stayed with me as a highlight of my time in Marrakech. A beggar woman, covered up, sitting in the corner with a small boy in her lap playing with his turquoise-colored plastic boots. Mom's hand reaches out to the passersby for spare change. She called out to her beautiful little girl who sat across the alley covered in rags. She must have been five or six years old, cheeks and nose were red from the cold. She perched on a worn-out wooden box, small tissue boxes for sale lined up neatly in front of her on a rag. I stood looking at her but she did not acknowledge me. She seemed to be in her own world, doing her own thing. Her right hand was gently moving. She drew a small circle in the dirt with a stick. Next to the circle laid a pile of small green leaves. With her tiny, cold hand she picked up one leaf at a time, arranged it, until soon the design of a flower took shape inside the circle. I was present and mesmerized, fixated on the hand of the little Buddha. Mom watched me, her eyes protecting her child. Just like the Buddhist monks creating their sand mandala only to let go of it in the wind as an act of impermanence, her creation would be gone by the street sweepers later that day. What becomes of her in the next decade? Would she be sitting on the other side of the alley where her mom is now, hand reaching to the passersby? Would a child be sitting in her lap with another child across the alley drawing a circle in the dirt while we make the next generation of the smartphones in the Silicon Valley? Time had slowed down for me; I am not sure how long I witnessed her work of art in its purest form. Picasso did a series of work on glass; a short film was made showing how he created, then destroyed them. On my way back to the town square, I placed a couple of coins in the mother's hand reaching out on the other side of the alley. She smiled at me as if she knew my name. We must have known each other in another life.

It must be noted that my initial paranoia never went away and for good reason. In most of my outings in Marrakech, I sensed I was being followed. Fortunately, I am a seasoned traveler who knows how to keep vigilant in unfamiliar places. Still, it becomes exhausting when always having to be on my guard, especially since I was traveling alone. A few times, I had to circle back to make sure I had been able to lose my follower. I was told these people would ask for a tip if I visited a tourist site, claiming they had shown me the way. I was not convinced by that argument. The characters following me were not ordinary looking Moroccans either. They dressed differently, in what appeared to be hand-me-down European clothing rather than Moroccan-style garb. Plus, they had a few old scars on their faces. The day before my departure, I visited one of the tourist attractions and was being followed, as usual. I asked one of the peddlers in charge of calling taxis why it was that I managed to get the attention of these followers. He responded, "You look like us, but do not dress like us. And you speak differently." That was his explanation of why I was followed. I was not convinced.

The Marathon: It was a perfect day to run in Marrakech; the desert sun showed its face in the last few miles of this fast and flat course. Unlike other marathon cutoff times, at kilometer 25 police were in charge and that meant only one thing: get on the bus if you missed the required cutoff. Once the race started, there were two groups: the fast ones who took off at a sprint and the not so fast, which was my group. After the first half of the race, the roads were open to traffic. Even with traffic control in most places, the drivers created their own sport by charging toward the runners to find out how close they could come without actually hitting us. Bikes, motorcycles and donkey carriages made sure they participated in the challenge. Sixteen kilometers into the race, I was pleased that a couple of kids were following me at the edge of the desert. One of them remarked on my nice shirt. Not long after that, a pack of kids ran behind me with a couple of them pulling on my shirt. As I turned, I noticed at least ten kids who were interested in my shirt. I stopped, smiled at them and, while gesturing to them to go back, I said "No." I began running again, concerned about the cut-off time at the 25th kilometer. They became even more aggressive. I picked up speed, but so did the kids; they could run fast in their worn-out slippers. I finally had to turn around and chase them away, while being watched by onlookers and other runners. I was happy when they were no longer in sight and no one was pulling on my shirt. Late in the race, other kids were lining the sidewalks and giving the runners high fives. A few had made a game of hitting the runners' hands pretty hard as they gave high fives in passing. When I got hit pretty hard and felt the tingle in my hand, I moved to the middle of the road.

At the end of the race, I could proudly proclaim, "All continents completed!" This self-created monkey was off my back.

Marathon Number 117
Marrakech Marathon
Morocco
January 2015

Ultramarathon - Also called ultra-distance or ultra-running, is any footrace longer than the traditional marathon length of 42.195 kilometers (26 mi 385 yd).
https://en.wikipedia.org/wiki/Ultramarathon

Ebola Virus Disease (EVD) - Is a rare and deadly disease in people and nonhuman primates. The viruses that cause EVD are located mainly in sub-Saharan Africa. People can get EVD through direct contact with an infected animal (bat or nonhuman primate) or a sick or dead person infected with Ebola virus.
https://www.cdc.gov/vhf/ebola/index.html

ISIS – Islamic State of Iraq and Syria, also known as ISIL (Islamic State of Iraq and the Levant), is a Sunni jihadist group with a particularly violent ideology that calls itself a caliphate and claims religious authority over all Muslims. It was inspired by al Qaida but later publicly expelled from it.
https://www.rand.org/topics/the-islamic-state-terrorist-organization.html#:~:text=ISIS%20(Islamic%20State%20of%20Iraq,later%20publicly%20expelled%20from%20it

Medina of Marrakesh - Founded in 1070–72 by the Almoravids, Marrakesh remained a political, economic and cultural center for a long period. Its influence was felt throughout the western Muslim world, from North Africa to Andalusia. It has several impressive monuments dating from that period: the Koutoubiya Mosque, the Kasbah, the battlements, monumental doors, gardens, etc. Later architectural jewels include the Bandiâ Palace, the Ben Youssef Madrasa, the Saadian Tombs, several great residences and Place Jamaâ El Fna, a veritable open-air theatre.
https://whc.unesco.org/en/list/331/

Bazaar - or souk, is a permanently enclosed marketplace or street where goods and services are exchanged or sold. The term bazaar originates from the Persian word bāzār. The term bazaar is sometimes also used to refer to the "network of merchants, bankers and craftsmen" who work in that area.
https://en.wikipedia.org/wiki/Bazaar

Jemaa el-Fnaa - (Arabic: ساحة جامع الفناء Sāḥat Jāmiʾ al-Fanāʾ, also Jemaa el-Fna, Djema el-Fna or Djemaa el-Fnaa) is a square and market-place in Marrakesh's medina quarter (old city). It remains the main square of Marrakesh, used by locals and tourists.
https://en.wikipedia.org/wiki/Jemaa_el-Fnaa

Gypsies - Also known as the Roma, are an Indo-Aryan people, traditionally nomadic itinerants living mostly in Europe, as well as diaspora populations in the Americas. The Romani are widely known in English by the exonym Gypsies (or Gipsies), which is considered by some Roma people to be pejorative due to its connotations of illegality and irregularity.
[63]https://en.wikipedia.org/wiki/Romani_people

Viber – Is a VoIP and instant messaging application with cross-platform capabilities that allows users to exchange audio and video calls, stickers, group chats, and instant voice and video messages.
https://whatis.techtarget.com/definition/Viber#:~:text=Viber%20is%20a%20VoIP%20and,instant%20voice%20and%20video%20messages.&text=The%20software%20also%20enables%20switching%20calls%20and%20chats%20between%20mobile%20and%20desktop

Visceral - Based on deep feeling and emotional reactions rather than on reason or thoughts.
https://dictionary.cambridge.org/us/dictionary/english/visceral

Impermanence - Called anicca (Pli) or anitya (Sanskrit), appears extensively in the Pali Canon as one of the essential doctrines of Buddhism. The doctrine asserts that all of conditioned existence, without exception, is "transient, evanescent, inconstant".
https://en.wikipedia.org/wiki/Impermanence#:~:text=Impermanence%2C%20called%20an-icca%20(P%C4%81li),transient%2C%20evanescent%2C%20inconstant%22

Marathon Cutoff Time - Typically, marathon cutoff times are around six hours. For example, athletes who run the Boston Marathon have six hours to complete the course. That means you›d have to average a pace of just under 14 minutes per mile.
https://www.verywellfit.com/how-strict-are-time-limits-in-races-2910929#:~:text=Typical-ly%2C%20marathon%20cutoff%20times%20are,under%2014%20minutes%20per%20mile

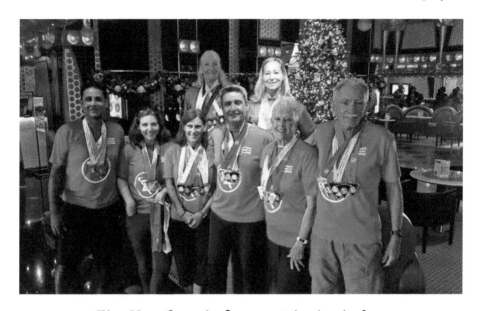

Five Marathons in five countries in six days

At the briefing dinner the night before the race, we were told that we would be running in a private golf resort the next day. This, by far, would be the highlight of the running trip, we would feel safe on private property. This was the fourth marathon of five in the Western Caribbean Challenge; five marathons, five countries in six days. We had started with a marathon in Miami, got on a cruise ship afterward, ran a marathon in Cozumel, Mexico the next day, then Belize before this one. The last race would be in the Cayman Islands. When we got to each port, we raced against time to finish and got back to the cruise ship for the next port. Our fellow passengers gave us strange looks when we disembarked at each port in our running gear. These were all self-supported runs. While taking refuge from the heat and buying water to replenish our supplies during the races, the shopkeepers told us we were crazy to run in the 90+ degree heat and high humidity so normal for their countries.

The stories read and told about Honduras were not comforting. The crime rates were high and tourists mostly avoided the country. In order not to be left behind by the cruise ship, we had to travel by bus to the resort and back. We were also told that we could run part of our race on the cruise ship track, which was about 1/8 mile long. I took advantage of the offer and went up to the top of the cruise ship in the early morning while it was dark. Soon enough, the rain and the wind picked up. I felt tired from the prior three races and lack of sleep, but the endorphins kicked in and I began to enjoy the short loops in the rain. I worked hard to remember the number of loops I ran so I could convert them to miles later.

Many of the runs we did on this trip were on the honor system since there were no aid stations or check points on the courses. While running on the small loop at the top of the cruise ship in the middle of the ocean in a heavy downpour, I noticed a handprint of a small child on a section of the loop near the ladder where I had climbed to get to the track. I did not pay too much attention until I returned back to the same spot and saw it again. I paused, ran and rushed to get to the same point on the third pass only to find the handprint on the track in the pouring rain. I was convinced that there had been a handprint on the track, but I did not think too much about it as I rushed to get to the meet-up place on the cruise ship so we could all take the small transport boats to shore.

We were to meet by the Christmas tree on the main deck, an obvious focal point as we were traveling in December. I must have sat near the tree forever and did not see anyone. Finally, I gave up and took the last boat in the rain to the shore where I found everyone waiting for me. Concerned, they asked me what happened, I told them I had waited but no one showed up. They said they had also waited for me but I did not show. Only later would I find out that I was not on the main deck where we were supposed to meet. I guess the boat had Christmas trees on every deck, enough to confuse me. The bus ride to the resort occurred mostly in haze coming in and out of something similar to sleep.

I could not recall the start of the race and only when the sun came up during the second loop of the race, did I find myself running. My brain must have shut down from the heat and exhaustion of the past few days. However, with temperature in the low 80's in the early part of the race, I found the run easier at the spectacular Princess Bay Resort on Isla of Roatan. I had fun being out there with new and old friends to run the race. On the hilly part of the course I could hear the cheer of friends and family from home in my mind.

In the next couple of days, the images of a handprint in the rain would come to mind but would soon fade. When I finally returned home after the last race, I could not sleep due to the time change. In the early hours of the morning while my family slept, I worked on my mail from the week before. When I got up to open the fridge for a bottle of water, I froze in my tracks. On the fridge door I saw a small child's handprint in red on a white piece of paper. I immediately backed off, thinking I was hallucinating. My curiosity got the best of me and I went back to look again; sure enough, there it was. I touched the edge of the paper carefully to make sure I was not imagining things. The paper was real and so was the image, but I still was not convinced.

The next morning when my wife woke up, I asked her to come to the kitchen with me to look at the paper with the handprint. I asked her if it was real and she responded, "Yes." She proceeded to tell me it was our five-year-old niece's school artwork and had been given to her a few days earlier. I concluded that the image on the cruise ship, albeit a hallucination, represented an undeniable connection to my family so far away. As far as not remembering the start of the race, I attributed it to an exhausted mind that had let go.

Marathon Number 139
Mahogany Bay Coral Marathon
Isla Roatan, Honduras
December 2015

Isle of Roatan - Roatán is an island in the Caribbean, about 65 kilometres off the northern coast of Honduras. It is located between the islands of Útila and Guanaja, and is the largest of the Bay Islands of Honduras. The island was formerly known in English as Ruatan and Rattan.
https://en.wikipedia.org/wiki/Roat%C3%A1n

Hallucination - are sensory experiences that appear real but are created by your mind. They can affect all five of your senses. For example, you might hear a voice that no one else in the room can hear or see an image that isn't real.
https://www.healthline.com/health/hallucinations#:~:text=Hallucinations%20are%20senso-ry%20experiences%20that,image%20that%20isn't%20real

Running in the City of Angels

The Los Angeles Marathon counted as my third consecutive day of running. I had done two marathons in the past two days in Long Beach, California. Needless to say, exhaustion crept in after driving to Los Angeles in a rush to get to the expo and pick up my race packet. Running consecutive marathons not only takes mental strength, but also requires training runs that create muscle memory for such racing. In the months leading up to these races, I incorporated long distance training runs on consecutive days, multiple times. In addition to paying attention to my diet, I made sure I had adequate rest and paid a visit to my doctor's office for a full physical and blood work. The evening before the Los Angeles race, I walked around the blocks near the hotel after dinner to help loosen up my legs. I iced my muscles and got a good night's rest. All these strategies helped me to wake up early and get to the start of the race at Dodger's Stadium.

I rode to the start line with a friend. By sunrise, I had settled under the pillars of the stadium trying to keep warm. I watched other runners come out of buses shivering in the morning cold. The unusual early morning chill in Los Angeles was unexpected and I did not have enough layers to stay warm. In big races such as the Los Angeles Marathon, nervous energy is always felt near the start, mixed with the smell of porta-potties. I could see the excitement of high schoolers in their bright green singlets as I tuned into the energy of the crowd near the start. They appeared to be restless and could not wait for the race to begin while they walked around nervously in small groups. Later, I learned that a few of the local school districts promoted this event for their students in an attempt to advocate for better health.

After walking around for a while in order to stay warm, I found refuge under the stairs leading up to the higher floors of the stadium. While watching the groups of young people walking around and bumping into one other, I spied a young lady dressed in a Cinderella costume with full make-up holding a small cage. She squeezed herself into a rare warm space across from me. Having nothing better to do, I focused on the contents of the cage. As I looked closer, I saw a tiny hamster wheel, a minuscule bowl of food, wood shavings and a little tube of water clipped to the side. The compact cage was white with pink trim but showed no sign of a hamster inside. The lady's costume matched the colors of the cage. She noticed my curious looks and I could not help but ask her if she was planning to take the cage with her for the race. To my surprise, she responded, "Yes." She went on to say that she had carried the cage with her pet hamster in other races. I asked her if it was safe to carry a cage for 26.2 miles and she felt it had never been a problem before, so why would it be one now? I finally spied the hamster hiding under the wood shavings. Just another one of the strange experiences one encounters while racing with big crowds.

Mixed with 25,000 runners and walkers, the energetic, nervous high schoolers in bright green singlets seemed to be commissioned to create chaos and injuries on the course. Early into the race I decided to call them angels after the City of Angels. Around mile two, one of them tripped the lady carrying her hamster. An hour earlier hamster lady had told me she would be carrying her "hammy" on her shoulder if carrying the cage became too uncomfortable for her. As she hit the pavement face down, she reached for the broken cage; hammy was nowhere to be found. A few runners helped her to her feet, and with a bloody face, she started calling out for her pet while the hoard of runners passed by.

The nervous energy of the angels set the tone for the run. They zigzagged across the course, ran into other runners, showered the crowd with Gatorade, tossed cups and bottles and came to a complete halt in front of others when they began to cramp up. As if a runner carrying a hamster was not enough of a strange experience for the day, these angels made sure to keep us all on our toes. Most of the angels came to rest at the medical tents at miles 16 and 18. A chosen few continued to create more hazards until they crossed the finish line.

Usually in big races, we run on the outskirts of the city and see the landmarks only from a distance. The Los Angeles Marathon took us past many of the top tourist destinations, starting at Dodger Stadium then going through West Hollywood, Beverly Hills, Rodeo Drive, Brentwood and finishing in Santa Monica. The course was not flat, as had been promised; hills rose up out there, especially in the early miles. I was glad to finish the race safely despite a few close calls with the mischievous angels.

Marathon Number 148
LA Marathon
February 2016

Race Packet - The packet typically includes your bib (the number you wear on the front of your body, usually pinned to your shirt) and may include a timing chip to attach to your shoe. The rest of what's in the packet is mostly pamphlets for other races, possibly some product samples or other swag, and the "free" T-shirt.
https://vitals.lifehacker.com/how-to-prepare-for-your-first-race-whether-it-s-a-5k-o-1735174408

Muscle Memory - the ability to repeat a specific muscular movement with improved efficiency and accuracy that is acquired through practice and repetition.
https://www.merriam-webster.com/dictionary/muscle%20memory

Cinderella - One resembling the fairy-tale Cinderella: such as. a : one suffering undeserved neglect. b : one suddenly lifted from obscurity to honor or significance.
https://www.merriam-webster.com/dictionary/Cinderella#:~:text=%3A%20one%20resembling%20the%20fairy%2Dtale,obscurity%20to%20honor%20or%20significance

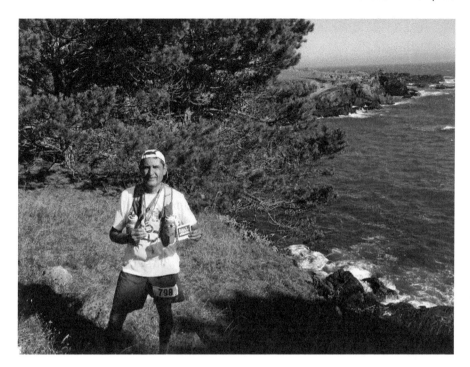

Ghost Runner

We were going to run a 50-kilometer race at Salt Point State Park in Jenner, California. The race site had described that we would run through ancient trails on the sacred land of "The Pomo" people. Since I had no knowledge of them, I did an online search and discovered

"The Pomo" are defined as indigenous people who lived around 1870 in northern California in a large territory bordered by the Pacific Coast to the west, extending inland to Clear Lake.

For me, race day started around 2:00 a.m. when I had to drive to my ultra-trail running friends' house 50 miles away from home which, unfortunately, was in the opposite direction of the race. I tried to go to bed earlier the night before but did not succeed. In order to stay awake during the dark drive, I blasted the music in the car and paid extra attention to the road. Many of the local trail races require an early morning start and I was used to it, but this one was much further away. Not only did I have to drive 50 miles to my friends' house, but we then had to drive another 80 miles to the starting line. Fortunately, a few of us were carpooling and my friend was going to drive us. He had had a few more hours of sleep than I and was an alert designated driver. I took the back seat of their car.

Once we left the San Francisco Bay Area, I started getting drowsy and took a nice nap before arriving at Salt Point State Park. The fog from the ocean shrouded the dirt parking lot when we pulled in. I was excited because, according to the race website, we were going to travel through time as we ran along the ancient trails of The Pomo people. We would also witness the wonders of the rugged coastline, sandstone cliffs, kelp-dotted coves, tide pools, Pygmy forests and, of course, the panoramic views. The course consisted of two loops going through the start/finish line near the scenic edge of the ocean. It totaled 54 kilometers with a 6,000-foot gain in elevation, a small detail I had overlooked in the fine print of the website. I liked the fact that this was going to be loops because, if I missed anything in the Pomo territory, I could catch it on the second loop.

We had a lot to do before the 7:00 a.m. start of the race and had to hustle. We stepped out of the car into the cold morning air. The first stop was to the start/finish line to get our bibs. Then we went back to the car to get our gear. A final mad dash to the bathrooms then we got to the start for the race briefing. By then the fog had burned off and sun warmed us up, but we still felt a nice cold breeze from the ocean.

The race director reminded us that we had to count on each other while we traversed the remote trails and help out if someone got injured or needed aid. Once the race started, one of the friends I carpooled with took off fast and I did not see much of him until the finish. I ran with my other friend. We had run over 50 trail races together and we had a compatible pace. She believes it is not about how you start the race, but how you finish it. Through the years I have bought into her belief; I have witnessed runners drop out of a race only a few miles before the finish. Besides injuries, mental breakdown can be a reason for some of the dropouts. Most runners are physically well-trained, but they overlook the need for mental training, especially on a technical trail, in the heat, with hills, such as this one.

Making our way toward the hills through the overgrown meadows, we made sure not to brush up against the poison oak bordering both sides of the narrow trail. A few runners passed us as we approached the first hill, but soon after we met up with them and power hiked the first steep hill together. Did I say hill? It really felt more like a vertical climb. As we say on the trails, there is an uphill for every downhill; however, that morning it was all about climbing before the trail finally leveled off at the top. The good part of the ascent was that we had some shade along the way and enjoyed the trees and vegetation surrounding the trail. During these beautiful scenes of nature, we got a chance to meet other runners in the race and joked about passing each other in a game of catch-up. Once on top of the hill, I found it hard to run and, looking down at my feet, I noticed sand. We were actually running in sand at that 3,000 foot high elevation!

We next encountered the Pygmy forest, a rare ecosystem featuring miniature trees and inhabited by small species of fauna such as rodents and lizards. Wikipedia tells me that these forests are usually located at high elevations, under conditions of sufficient air humidity but poor soil. We saw a variety of trees here but the special treat for me was running through dwarf redwood trees that were over 100 years old. It seemed surreal to see grown trees shorter than me. Due to the technical nature of the trail, with the hidden tree roots, I found it difficult to fully appreciate the beauty of the forest. I had to look down and stay focused on 2-3 feet ahead of my steps on the trail.

After a few long miles we entered an open space ringed with a lush green forest of tall trees and fern covered groves. The climate cooled and a sweet smell hung in the air. It felt strange to go first through a forest of short trees and now tall ones. We ran through it quickly before arriving at a fire road that dropped down toward a school, we could see a mile below. We were taken aback to see a yellow school bus at that elevation, so close to such beautiful forests and far away from the sea. We could see young musicians in their black pants and red shirts carrying their instruments into the school. My friend and I suspected that there was an event or a rehearsal going on, but wondered who would come see them considering the remote location of the school?

As we dropped down a steep rocky path, we had to bring our attention back to the trail. We were happy and playful while we jumped over small rocks and let gravity take us down toward the ocean. We got glimpses of water in a few spots before we finally started running on the cliff edge next to the sea. The ocean view, with the breeze fanning us, was refreshing and the beauty of the meadows, strewn with colorful flowers, gave us the second wind we needed to finish the first loop.

Next to the timing mat at the start/finish area, we stopped at the aid station. We always joked about not sitting on the chair at the aid stations since getting up is a monumental task. This day we saw a runner hunched over in the chair holding his head. A closer look revealed his bloodied elbows and knees. The blood was still dripping from his knees as he had lost a lot of skin. The medics had started attending to him. Scenes like this on trail races are always disturbing since it can happen to any of us no matter how careful we try to be, especially when there are stretches when we do not see anyone for miles.

When I passed the timing mat and glanced at the timer with bright red numbers on it, I let out a sigh of relief. We had made the cut off and had plenty of time to complete the second loop. My friend and I did not spend too much time there, so as soon as we got our water bottles filled up, we were on our way toward the hills. I had grabbed a cup of water as we left the aid station and took a big gulp, but the water went down the wrong pipe. I came to a halt not too far from the timing mat and started coughing and choking. Between coughs, I would look up to see my friend's concerned face. I was in trouble. I bent over and tried to get the water out. It took a lot of coughing and hacking in order to get some relief. Fortunately, my friend stayed with me during this ordeal. Once I could breathe again, we began the climb up the first hill of the loop we had started earlier in the morning. I wondered if all that coughing and choking was going to have any impact during the rest of my run. With an irritated throat and a light headache, I pushed up the hills and made my way back to the Pygmy forest.

We were enjoying the trail in the Pygmy forest, my friend pacing a few steps ahead of me, when I heard a sound in the woods to my right. I turned to investigate, and I saw a small barefoot guy with short loose black pants and a long white robe running parallel to me in the trees. His long hair was flying while he ran smoothly, not on the ground but seemingly in the air. A big smile on his face showed his bright white teeth. It appeared as though he was looking straight at me. I kept watch on my friend ahead of me and the runner to my right. I am not sure how long we ran before my friend said something about the poison oak close to our legs. We both came to a halt. She noticed my blank look and wanted to know if I was okay. I asked her if she had seen the guy in the woods who was running with us before we stopped. She had a big smile on her face and said, "We have not had any company for the past few miles." I carefully considered this as I took a sip from my water bottle. I was puzzled. She explained that I must have been hallucinating. I was not convinced but trusted her judgment. Looking at the dense wood to my right, I realized it was nearly impossible for anyone to run there. I did not know what to think of what I had seen. While we continued our run, I tried to stay closer to my friend.

We came to the lush forest again with the sweet smell in the air. This time we heard the beautiful sound of a cello. I remembered the school bus and the musicians we had seen earlier and thought maybe I could hear them playing down in the school. As the sound became stronger, I noticed a guy with black pants and a red shirt playing cello. He sat on a tree trunk surrounded by ferns. I could not see his face as his head was down and he seemed to be focused on his performance. I stopped. Since I was ahead of my friend this time, I looked back at her and she asked, "Why did you stop?" I pointed to the guy and said, "Look!" Now it was her turn to be puzzled. I asked, "Can you hear the music?" and she said, "What music?....not again!" I knew what she meant and, just to make sure I was not hallucinating again, I walked toward the guy. He lifted his head and looked at me. I went close enough to touch his shirt. He stopped playing and asked, "What are you doing?" I asked him if he was for real and he gave me a strange look. I shook my head, returned to the trail and continued running.

A mile down the hill, we saw the musicians with black pants and red shirts around the school bus; that made me feel better. I looked at my friend and she had a huge smile on her face. I asked her, "Was the guy we saw earlier for real?" She said, "Yes." She also said, "That was a great opportunity to mess with your head. The guy must have climbed up the hill with his instrument to find a quiet place in the woods to play his cello." I was not convinced. The hike was about a mile up a steep hill and his cello looked pretty heavy. We did not talk anymore about the two guys I saw up in the forests as we made our way to the finish line.

During a busy day at work a couple of days after the race, I suddenly remembered the guy who was running with me in the woods. I stopped my work and went to the race website to read more about where we had run. I was reminded that we were running on The Pomo's sacred land. I started researching about The Pomo. Suddenly, I froze. On my screen appeared a fuzzy picture of the guy who ran with me in the woods that day.

Marathon and Ultra 163
Salt Point 50k
Salt Point State Park
July 2016

Clear Lake – is a natural freshwater lake in Lake County in the U.S. state of California, north of Napa County and San Francisco. It is the largest natural freshwater lake wholly within the state, with 68 square miles (180 km2) of surface area. At an age of 2.5 million years, it is the oldest lake in North America. It is the latest lake to occupy a site with a history of lakes stretching back at least 2,500,000 years.
https://en.wikipedia.org/wiki/Clear_Lake_(California)

Salt Point State Park - Located on the rugged California coastline about 90 miles north of San Francisco on State Highway One, and 8 miles north of Fort Ross State Historic Park. The shoreline of the 6,000-acre park features rocky promontories, such as Salt Point, that juts out into the Pacific Ocean. There are two campgrounds and more than 20 miles of hiking trails in the park.
http://www.saltpoint.org/

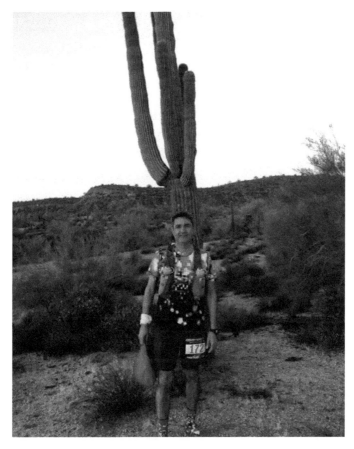

The Sonoran Desert

The 100K (62.2 mile) race called the Javelina Jundred took place under Arizona's hot sun in the Sonoran Desert at McDowell Mountain Regional Park. This race had been on my radar for a while. I traveled with ultra-friends Fran, who would run with me, and her husband Ray, who was going to pace us on the last part of the race. We had booked an early morning flight out of San Francisco, California to Phoenix, Arizona. We got to the airport shortly after midnight and slept in our sleeping bags near the gate to await our flight.

On their website, the race director had taken pride in emphasizing that 50% of the participants usually drop out of the race in both distances of 100 miles and 100 kilometers. He warned us about heat stroke in the daytime and hypothermia at night in the desert. Just thinking about half of the participants dropping out kept me concerned as we drove to the start of the race to check in and get our tents (yes, we would be camping). The tents were set up in a makeshift campsite on the dusty desert near the start line. Getting out of the car, in the afternoon heat of the desert, felt like walking into a furnace. We checked in quickly. I dropped my bag in my tiny tent and looked around to make sure I did not have the company of any desert creatures. We could not wait to return to the air-conditioned car, head back to town, pick up our bib numbers and race gear at the race expo, and eat in an air-conditioned burger place. We saw a few familiar faces at the expo, and they were clearly nervous about this race.

We made a trip to the nearby grocery store to pick up race food, ice, drinks and a Styrofoam ice chest. As we unloaded the car at the campsite, the ice chest broke apart upon landing. I stood and watched how fast all the ice spread onto the dirt and promptly melted into the ground. Many years ago, in Eastern Europe's harsh winter, my brother and I stood on a sidewalk and watched how quickly water turned into ice when the temperature dropped to negative16 degrees Centigrade. The polar opposite experiences of watching the interaction of water and earth were surreal. In the flimsy ice chest, that ice would not have lasted anyways, I thought while I gathered the broken pieces and walked toward my tent.

After sunset the weather turned cool and I had to put on another layer of clothing. I enjoyed being in the desert with other ultrarunners. In an open space outside of the tent area, vendors sold pizza, snacks, and to my amazement they had set up cash registers with credit card machines under their canopies. While eating a slice of pizza, I sat on a rock and watched a documentary on a makeshift screen about an ultrarunner. The cold seeped into the tent around midnight and I had to add a few more layers. The noise in the campsite and jitters of the race ahead made it difficult to get a good night's sleep.

The 100-mile runners started an hour ahead of us. I made sure to wake up early, before the sunrise, so I could cheer them on when they began. Later we would see some of them dropping out of the race due to the extreme heat. A quick snack followed by stretching and we were ready to start the race. The sun rose over the Sonoran Desert and, at 7:00 a.m., the temperature already seemed as if it were mid-afternoon.

The race consisted of three loops of trails. I was thrilled to see the Tarahumara runners from the Copper Canyon in Mexico lined up with us at the start, complete with their colorful costumes and sandals. They are some of the world's best distance runners and the subject of the popular book "Born to Run". A few of them ended up dropping out. It may have had to do with their poor placement in the race that would have deprived them of their goal of victory. They are such excellent endurance runners that I do not believe the heat or elevation gain bothered them much.

The temperature was supposed to reach the high 90s Fahrenheit and it already felt pretty hot when we started the race. Fran reminded me that it is how we finish the race that counts, not the way we start. Soon we were going at an easy pace with eyes glued on the trail to make sure we did not step on any desert creatures. I found the race to be extremely well organized with fully stocked aid stations in the most remote places. Coyotes and tarantulas were plentiful, while the rattlesnakes and scorpions stayed off the trails. However, as the temperature rose to 103 degrees Fahrenheit, runners started dropping like flies due to heat stroke. The emergency crews got busy. We even witnessed a Medivac helicopter making circles above our heads, eventually raising the dust from the desert floor while it landed ahead of us to rescue a downed injured runner.

On the first loop of 23 miles, even I became part of an ad hoc emergency crew. We climbed up a hill around mile 19 and saw a runner sitting on the side of the trail with her head down and a few runners trying to help. A quick assessment confirmed she suffered from heat stroke and had no fluids left in her water bottle. I poured half of my water over her head and asked her name. She responded but had difficulty conversing. She did not want to stand up. When I asked her about her children, a spark came to her eyes and then she had a willingness to try getting up to her feet. For the next four miles of the loop, I made sure she stayed well hydrated by giving her all my water and electrolyte drink in small sips. The other runners who had stopped to help her stayed with us as we headed to the race headquarters and the medical tent. I was dehydrated but none of the accompanying runners had been willing to share their fluids. Once we checked into the medical tent, she gave me a big hug and I told the medic they might consider administering intravenous fluids right away. While she was being hooked up to monitors and questioned by the medics, I told them to take good care of her. Apparently, I did not look good upon arrival as one of the medics asked me if I had been hydrating. I told him yes, with the exception of the last four miles walking. He offered to take my vitals, but I told him that I was behind in my pace and needed to get out there. A hundred yards away, after I filled my bottles, I sat on a chair by the main aid station and Fran managed to find me. I had to sit for a while as I felt dizzy and could not move. With food and drinks, eventually I felt better, and we were back in the desert on another loop. When I went back to the medic tent after the second loop to get checked out for a blister, they told me that I was like a ghost who brought in the sick runner, then vanished. They once again said that I did not look good and offered me an emergency check-up, but I refused their offer.

During the run, we came across runners sitting on the side of the dirt trail being tended to by the paramedics. We ran into runners going the wrong way and they were too disoriented to listen to our directions. At the next aid station, a group of runners with defeated looks waited for a ride after dropping out of the race. I had brought small Ziploc bags and got them filled with ice at every aid station. I put them under my hat and in less than half a mile all the ice had melted. I would then drink the warm water from the bag.

They called one aid station in the middle of the desert "Jackass Junction". It had a disco party theme with a dance floor and strobe light. The loud music could be heard several hundred feet before and after the aid station. A few runners took time to stay around and dance until the volunteers kicked them out. After sundown, the weather got cooler and I added on a light layer to make sure not to suffer from hypothermia. The night desert was full of stars and we saw the 100-mile runners doing their loops in the opposite direction. Even the race director was freed up to do a loop and, as course marshal, check on runners. Our mood improved since we knew the finish line lay a few miles away from our last aid station. At one point on the way back, I thought I saw the runner who we had helped to the medic tent but could not be sure. A few weeks after the race, the heat stroked lady I helped rescue found me on Facebook to thank me and tell me that she had actually finished the race despite her setbacks. I found a new tough friend and was relieved to learn that she was fine.

As arranged, Fran's husband Raymond met up with us to pace us on the last loop. He had suffered an injury on a previous race and decided to volunteer all day at the headquarters' aid station. On the last loop, about seven miles into pacing us in the dark, he fell off the trail on the side of a small hill and aggravated his injury. He could no longer run but assured us he would be fine. Fran decided to stay with him so that they could walk together to the next aid station. I continued the run.

After 16 hours and two minutes it felt good to run and run fast. I passed a lot of runners and made a short stop for water at the last aid station before the finish line. A couple of runners sat at the aid station waiting for their friends before they ventured out in the pitch dark. I was not comfortable to be on my own for the last few miles but did not want to lose precious time. During the final 3.7 miles of the race, I passed a few runners and saw a couple of 100 milers. Then it was the darkness with not a soul in sight. The desert loomed magically, especially at night with no light pollution. I turned off my headlamp so I could enjoy the moon and the stars in the silence of the desert. I made sure to stay on the trail and paid close attention to all the sounds around me. A couple of miles before the finish line, I heard stealthy footsteps and turned my headlamp back on. The light reflected in the eyes of creature and made some shadows visible. As I switched my headlamp to a brighter light, I saw a pack of coyotes all around me and one of them stood his ground right in front me. At that moment I hoped to see runners on the trail, but no one showed up from either direction. I shouted and ran hard toward the one that blocked the trail ahead of me. It disappeared fast, but I could see that he had marked the trail. The other eyes in the dark disappeared with the lead coyote. Even though I had been running for hours and now found myself all alone out there in the pitch black around 1:00 a.m. in the desert, I knew that encounter was no hallucination. I looked around, found a long stick and carried it until I heard the music of the finish line and saw the lights of the race headquarters. I felt a huge relief as I went through the finish line just after 2:00 a.m..

I did not stay around to wait for Fran and her husband. I saw them the next morning by the showers on the other side of the campsite. Instead, after a few bites of the finish line food, I crashed in my tent and heard someone suffering from hypothermia nearby. They were calling the emergency medic while I fell into a deep sleep.

Marathon and Ultra Number171
Javelina Jundred Kilometer
Fountain Hills, AZ
October 2016

Sonoran Desert – The Sonoran Desert is a North American desert and ecoregion which covers large parts of the Southwestern United States in Arizona and California and of Northwestern Mexico in Sonora, Baja California, and Baja California Sur. It is the hottest desert in Mexico. It has an area of 260,000 square kilometers.
https://en.wikipedia.org/wiki/Sonoran_Desert

Heat Stroke – Is a condition caused by your body overheating, usually as a result of prolonged exposure to or physical exertion in high temperatures. This most serious form of heat injury, heatstroke, can occur if your body temperature rises to 104 F (40 C) or higher. The condition is most common in the summer months.
https://www.webmd.com/a-to-z-guides/heat-stroke-symptoms-and-treatment

Hypothermia – Is a medical emergency that occurs when your body loses heat faster than it can produce heat, causing a dangerously low body temperature. Normal body temperature is around 98.6 F (37 C). Hypothermia (hi-poe-THUR-me-uh) occurs as your body temperature falls below 95 F (35 C).
https://www.mayoclinic.org/diseases-conditions/hypothermia/symptoms-causes/syc-20352682#:~:text=Hypothermia%20is%20a%20medical%20emergency,95%20F%20(35%20C)

Tarahumara Runners – The Rarámuri or Tarahumara are a group of indigenous people of the Americas living in the state of Chihuahua in Mexico. They are renowned for their long-distance running ability.
https://en.wikipedia.org/wiki/Rar%C3%A1muri#:~:text=The%20Rar%C3%A1muri%20or%20Tarahumara%20are,their%20long%2Ddistance%20running%20ability

Medivac – Is a service that provides medical care to injured patients while they are being transported from the scene of an accident to a hospital. This word is created from "medical" and "evacuation".
https://www.collinsdictionary.com/us/dictionary/english/medivac#:~:text=Medivac%20is%20a%20service%20that,%22medical%22%20and%20%22evacuation%22

Intravenous Fluid – Usually shortened to 'IV' fluids, are liquids given to replace water, sugar and salt that you might need if you are ill or having an operation, and can't eat or drink as you would normally. IV fluids are given straight into a vein through a drip.
https://www.nice.org.uk/guidance/ng29/ifp/chapter/what-are-intravenous-fluids#:~:text=Intravenous%20fluids%20(usually%20shortened%20to,a%20vein%20through%20a%20drip

Course Marshall - Course marshals oversee key points on the race course (turns, intersections, etc…) to insure that runners are directed along the race route, and to insure that runners may proceed safely, free of vehicle traffic and other preventable dangers.
https://medium.com/@CARArunsGreg/race-directors-a-case-for-course-marshals-42dec8fd-bc87

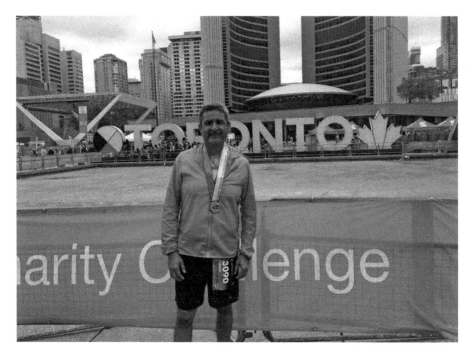

Heart of Hearts

I started the trail marathon on a hot day in the summer of 2017 at Lake Chabot in Castro Valley, California. The early morning temperature read in the low 70s, but soon became 20 degrees hotter. As the race progressed, we started climbing the hills. On the second loop, around mile 16, I found a little bit of shade to sit down on the side of a steep hill overlooking the lake. I stopped there because, climbing up the hill with temperatures in the high 90's, my heart pounded as if it were ready to fly out of my chest. This unfamiliar feeling concerned me. Because of the heat and hills, a few runners had abandoned the marathon and settled for the half marathon, dropping out at the start of the second loop. I could not see anyone either behind or ahead of me. I took a few deep breaths and my mind raced. I wondered if I was suffering from heat stroke. The next aid station was on top of the hill, another three miles up a steep climb. With no one around, I worried about my safety for the first time in nearly 200 marathons and ultras.

I decided I must follow up with a specialist because of this new scare. Not that I had not been trying. The past few months found me in and out of my doctor's office complaining about a shortness of breath that occurred a few miles into my races. I insisted on an EKG and Stress Test; he performed the tests and the results were normal. My doctor said everything seemed fine with my heart, that I should train harder and continue running. I took his advice, but in almost every race I encountered trouble a few miles from the start.

Another time I went back to my doctor to complain about oxygen deprivation during races. Previously, he had discovered an H. Pylori bacterial infection in my stomach. Because I was taking a high dosage of antibiotic for this problem, my doctor felt that my breathing had to do with gas build-up that pushed through my esophagus during running. Even during my training runs, I experienced shortness of breath. I kept on pushing hard, convinced it had to do with my conditioning. My body rejected the strenuous workouts and I consistently ended up out of breath, gasping for air on my neighborhood sidewalks and holding a tree or a pole for balance. After catching my breath, I would continue to make frequent stops before finishing my runs.

I had read every article I could find on-line about sudden death in marathons and shortness of breath while running. Nothing conclusive emerged as my research continued. I had troubleshot everything I could think of, but my unusual heartbeat was new and that concerned me. When no one showed up on the trail that hot day, I had no choice but to get up and keep going. A part of me wanted to finish the race, as I have been conditioned to do, so I pushed on up the steep hill instead of going down toward the finish line. Having run this race a few times in the past, I knew that the winding trail crossed a paved road about a mile up. There I might be able to flag down a car for help. I kept hydrated while struggling to climb up and took a few more breaks before getting to the road. I stood out there in the heat and sipped on water, but no cars passed by. Eventually I gave up and, as my heartbeat started getting back to normal, gained enough confidence to hike up the next hill where I knew an aid station would be. The aid tent sat by the main road and the trail continued on the other side. When I arrived, a sheriff's car pulled up, two policemen jumped out, opened the back door and let out a guy in handcuffs. The scene we witnessed seemed so surreal that both the volunteer at the aid station and I looked at each other without any words being exchanged. How fortuitous. I had looked for help earlier and here were two cops right in front of me. Before I could say anything, they unlocked the handcuffs, gave the guy his T-shirt, then jumped back in the car and took off.

There have been times in some tough races when I have hallucinated. This time I did not know if what I had just witnessed was for real, until the guy walked up to the volunteer and asked for water. We did not ask him who he was and what had happened. I just knew I did not want to stay around for much longer to find out. I filled my water bottle, took a few pieces of boiled potatoes and asked the volunteer if there were any other runners ahead of me. He said most had long passed and he did not think there would be anyone behind me, but he would wait another half an hour before packing up to leave. He told me the next aid station could be found 4.5 miles down the trail in the wilderness. My new goal became making it there and the downhill on the other side of road helped me make up some lost time. While running, I ate the potatoes, washed them down with water and felt better. The only things that existed for me in that moment were the heat, the hills and the never-ending trail.

On this particular day, while I drowned in the beauty surrounding me, I did not realize the miles that passed. These are the best miles in races; I call it meditative running. A volunteer at the next aid station in the woods greeted me, happy to see someone. I refilled my water and he told me I had another 5 kilometers to the finish beyond the hill in front of us. My heart no longer pounded and my breath returned to normal. I felt healthy. A slow jog up the hill turned into a downhill run before two lost hikers stopped to ask me for directions. I could only offer them water since I did not know the campsite they were looking for. Going down around the lake, shade covered the paved trail and a few people hiked up toward the hills. My concern for myself temporarily vanished and I enjoyed my run to the finish line.

My goal for 2017 was to run at least one marathon each week and the "UltraSignup" trail racing calendar detailed runs within 200 miles of home that offered me perfect opportunities. These trail marathons also provided good training for a 100-mile race I wanted to do at the end of the year. Halfway through 2017, my breathing problems caused me to be unsure if I could make it to the start of that race. However,

I stayed with the goal of at least a marathon distance race each week and completed the 100-mile race in Arizona at the end of the year as I had scheduled, albeit with breathing difficulties.

The doctor visits continued regularly in 2017 and 2018 with the same complaints. More tests, including multiple EKGs, Stress Tests, Ultrasounds and blood work-ups, were performed. According to my doctor, specialists and the cardiologists, the results did not indicate any heart issues. I was given a heart monitor to wear for 48 hours and it showed no abnormality. A family history of my dad having a heart attack in his early 50's and my mom dying of heart disease had no impact on my arguments with the specialists and cardiologists, primarily because their test results indicated I had no heart disease. Instead, the doctors' attention focused on allergies and asthma, so breathing tests were scheduled. All tests showed no abnormalities.

I visited the Emergency Room twice after trail races in 2017. On one occasion, while driving to work one Monday after a race the day before, I experienced the sensation of a heart attack. I went directly to the Emergency Room at Kaiser Hospital and described all the symptoms of a heart attack to the nurse. She immediately got me admitted, put an IV in my arm and hooked me up to many devices in preparation for another CT scan. I had requested and argued with the cardiologist in charge about getting this scan because he thought I should not be exposed to any more radiation. As I lay in the Intensive Care Unit waiting for my CT Scan test results, the paramedics brought in a patient loaded with monitors and put him next to me. The same cardiologist who had visited me upon admission, showed up on the Code Blue call. After examining the patient, he turned to me and said this person was suffering from a heart attack. As I recall clearly, he told me there was nothing wrong with my heart. A few hours later, after that patient got wheeled into the operating room for an emergency by-pass, they gave me a few Tylenol, told me I had pulled my trapezoid muscle and should be able to get back to running in a few days.

On Labor Day weekend of 2017, I volunteered at a trail race aid station in the Bay Area on a relatively warm day. I enjoyed cheering on the runners while making sure they hydrated sufficiently when they passed by our aid station. An hour into the race, while the runners were making their loops for the half marathon, I saw a younger runner coming toward our table clearly struggling. As he got close, he suddenly collapsed. I ran toward him, put him in a safe position and, having been certified in first aid, jumped into action by asking his name and if he knew where he was. He tried talking but did not make any sense. This spelled trouble, so I called out for help and asked others to call 911. With the help of a few runners, we moved the aid station canopy overhead to try to keep him cool. He began to struggle for breath and lost his pulse. We started CPR and took turns. The race director came by and dropped off a portable automated external defibrillator (AED) machine that we hooked up right away and followed its voice command. At one point, a runner stopped in a panic to tell us that the man was his brother. We asked him to stick around to provide information to the medic. While witnessing the entire CPR scene, he totally lost it. Others then had to tend to him while he had a panic attack. Due to the remoteness of the trail, the medic took nearly an hour to arrive and take over from us. It felt like forever. After a couple of days, I found out through the race director that the young runner had survived the ordeal and would be released from the hospital soon. These experiences were unsettling for me since I still did not know the source of my own breathing difficulties.

In my next races in 2017 and 2018, the shortness of breath showed up a lot earlier. My concern kept sending me back to my doctors only to be told all was good with my heart. They now focused more on food allergies and other possible issues. At one point, my doctor thought he would feel better if my vocal chords were checked. The specialist visit consisted of the insertion of a tiny camera through my nose and into my throat, which caused a most unpleasant severe gag reflex. Other tests included a biopsy of my stomach lining to make sure there were "no serious issues" as my doctor put it. I did not know what to expect when they wheeled me into the operating room under a bright light and told me to count down to 1 from 50. I began and, just as I was getting drowsy, the physician in charge asked me where I was born. When I told him Iran, he proceeded to say that he had been seeing a lot of stomach cancer in Middle Eastern men lately. That certainly was not a comforting statement to hear prior to going under. Before I could respond to him about how I felt about his comment, I was out. They inserted a tube with a camera down my throat. This test confirmed the H.Pylori bacteria; a diagnosis I mentioned earlier that had no relation to my breathing problems. This took my physician further down the wrong path of treatment.

I continued reading about sudden death in marathons across the nation and was concerned about my own health. When I crossed the finish line in one of the local trail marathons in the spring of 2018, the race director informed me that a runner had died of a heart attack on the trail while running the half marathon that day. Other runners took turns and administered CPR for about 45 minutes but, when the medics showed up, it was too late. He had traveled from out of town for the race and his family waited for him at the finish line. I can only imagine their despair for the loss of their loved one.

These stories and experiences shook me to the core; however, my doctor and cardiologist kept insisting that my heart was fine and I should not be concerned. No matter how hard they tried, they could not convince me. I remained determined to find the source of my breathing troubles in races because I had no symptoms when I was not running. I continued to race and struggle; I also became cautious and paid much closer attention to my body.

By now, over a year had passed since I first began experiencing symptoms. I had more testing in 2018 and I continued running marathons and ultras. Breathing difficulties and chest tightness persevered when I ran but got better 8-10 miles into each race. Sometimes, I would struggle at the end of the race, but still managed to place in my age group. I continued to visit my doctor and cardiologist after my races. I insisted on getting more tests of my heart and, as more CT scans followed, my doctor again expressed concern about the radiation exposure and discouraged me from requesting any more.

An opportunity showed up to run the Toronto Marathon in October of 2018, so I signed up. My lower back and hips were giving me grief and I visited a specialist and my chiropractor for relief. I missed a few races and wondered if I would make it to Toronto. I took it easy with races in early autumn and added extra hours of yoga to rehab my lower back so I could travel, stay with relatives in Canada and run the marathon.

In Toronto, two days before the race, I went out in the cold October morning for a short run to check my breathing and lower back. As I climbed a small hill toward the mansions at the end of the street, the neighborhood of Vaughan shone brightly with colorful autumn leaves while home security cameras followed my every step. Unfortunately, less than a mile into the run, my chest felt tight and I had difficulty breathing. I took it easy for the rest of the run and focused on the trees and the elegant surroundings. I was a little worried about the strict cut-off time of the race. I tried not to think of it much and enjoyed the sights, family and food. After the expo the day before the race, I drove to Niagara Falls with my relatives, but the journey took longer than expected due to heavy traffic in and out of Toronto. I was exhausted by the time we returned in the late evening before the race.

By the time I got dropped off at the start in the early morning on race day, I felt tired from the cumulative effect of all the traveling. I found shelter at a downtown hotel with a lot of other runners and stayed warm until the race started. The excited energy of the crowd, mixed with anxiety, are always the fascinating highlights of distance racing for me. The nervous energy, combined with fear at the start of big races, has its own scent. Once the race starts, the scent evaporates as runners focus on their own universes. When we lined up at the start of the race, I wiped away the memory of my breathing difficulties during the run a few days earlier.

Everything began smoothly enough but, a kilometer into the race, my chest got tight and I could not breathe. Typically, in other road races, it had been 2-3 miles before the breathing problems started. The race began on a wide street and I had enjoyed my pace moving with the crowd. When the breathing problem started, I jumped off to the sidewalk, bent down and tried to catch my breath. When I felt better, I joined the crowd back on the street only to experience difficulty breathing again. Eventually, I pulled to the right side and started fast-walking with a purpose. The goal for the day had changed. I would finish the race safely, get back home to see my doctor and get to the bottom of this nagging problem. After the eight-kilometer mark, I felt better and started a jog that turned into a run. For distraction, I tried counting the number of runners that I passed, but soon got bored.

Next, I did a self-evaluation to make sure everything was working well. I made up for some of the lost time but came to halt at the 35-kilometer mark. Looking at my watch, I calculated my pace and realized I had plenty of time to walk the remaining seven kilometers for a safe finish. I finished the race with a little over half an hour to spare from the cut-off.

On the flight home, I strategized how to have a different conversation with my physician so that we could find the source of my breathing problems. My ultimate goal consisted of getting a referral to a different cardiologist who could order a heart scan called a Coronary Calcium Test. I had heard about this test from a friend a few months back and had done some research on-line about it. A score of 1 to 99 indicates calcium is beginning to accumulate and score over 100 suggests taking statins to control the cholesterol level.

My doctor happened to be on vacation, so I received an appointment with his assistant, a young physician who appeared to have just graduated from medical school. She prided herself in reviewing my chart before entering the exam room and tried hard to impress. However, our conversation went nowhere. Twice I sent her out to get me a referral for a different cardiologist who could order the Coronary Calcium Test. We had a bit of a back and forth, combined with my threat of not leaving until I got the referral. They granted me a phone appointment with a new cardiologist and, after half an hour of arguing with him, he ordered the test. After so much time and frustration, I had learned to be an advocate for my own health, but I still had more battles to fight.

To add insult to injury, during the preparation for the Coronary Calcium Test, a power struggle ensued between two nurses over the insertion of a line into my vein so that the contrast dye could be injected for the scan. Each of them claimed to be the expert on the procedure, but neither seemed to be having much success. By the time I lay under the CT Scan, their multiple attempts and arguments had exhausted me. The presence of one of the nurses, who insisted on trying to correct everyone in the room, became irritating. A new cardiologist, fresh out of school, introduced himself and said he would be present and would share the test results with me immediately after the scan. With no confidence in the staff surrounding me, I stayed nervous throughout the test. Afterwards, the cardiologist was nowhere to be found. After a few phone messages, I finally located him three days later. He informed me that my calcium number was elevated and an angioplasty needed to be done in order to find out what could be causing the high number. According to him, the number was supposed to be between 100-300, mine had registered 835.

In the next few days, I fought with everyone in Kaiser's Cardiology Department to make sure I would not be under the care of that particular cardiologist, nor would I allow him to be present during the procedure. Eventually, I got assigned to the cardiologist that I had originally requested. At the pre-op with my preferred cardiologist I asked all of my questions, including what side effects and risks to expect. Apparently, death is a possible risk of an angioplasty. He also informed me that, if a blockage were detected, they would insert a stent while I was under the knife. I gave my written consent.

My wife took me for the outpatient procedure on November 11, 2018. After learning about death being a possible risk, she became alarmed. I had failed to share that piece of information with her. While they prepared me for the operation, she mustered up the courage to ask me, "What if things go wrong?" I informed her that all of our affairs were in order and she would be making all of the decisions. We joked about "no vegetable," meaning no life support if I ended up in a vegetative state. When they rolled me into the operating room, the nurse told me that I would get the "good stuff." I remained half-awake throughout the operation, but the clock somehow moved faster, I blamed it on the "good stuff." I recall the surgeon telling me I had a 95% blockage in my right artery and they were proceeding with a stent. I gave a thumbs-up and felt the balloon in my vein just before they injected more of the "good stuff" into my system. Immediately after the procedure, I felt relieved because I could finally take in a deep breath. In recovery, they told me another 90% blockage existed on the left side of my heart but, because of the location, they were not able to put in a stent. With half of my heart fixed, the blockage remains. I have been told by my cardiologist that the condition is not life threatening. Kaiser's medical system nearly killed me but, because I learned to advocate strongly for myself, it finally saved me.

Post-operation required rehabilitation, which meant I had to attend a class session in person. Having taught at a university for over 25 years, I was shocked when I entered my rehab class because the classroom in the hospital looked more like a recovery room and there were not many participants. Before it began, we had blood pressure tests administered by the nurses present. After introductions, I learned that some of the others had had open-heart surgery with multiple bypasses. It became obvious to me that many had suffered a major trauma. A couple of the students shared their stories in-depth, thinking "physical rehab" meant a psychological therapy session. One of the nurses conducting the class struggled to keep order among the constant interruptions from the participants; this amused and entertained me. A lot of questions arose since we were all charting new territory with our repaired hearts. One of the patients asked when it would be safe to have sex again. The nurse responded, "When you can climb three flight of stairs without any shortness of breath." I could not help myself, I turned to the person who asked the question and asked him if he lived in a three-story building. The nurse puzzled at my joke, especially when I asked her why his partner could not come to the first floor instead of him climbing the stairs. I tried to add humor to these serious conversations, but my comments were not welcomed.

On a follow-up with my cardiologist, I asked him if I could run; he said I should be fine. A week after the procedure I did a few short runs and everything seemed to be working well, so I signed up for a local trail race. Forty days after my stent procedure, I ran a trail marathon. I chose that particular race with care in order to make sure that, if I got in trouble, I would have access to help. I packed my medication and, for the first time, took my phone with me. The course consisted of two loops with minimal elevation gain. I took it easy and prepared to call it quits if I ran into trouble. I am happy to report that I did not have to take walking breaks to catch my breath, as I had done for the last couple of years. I stayed at 70% of my efforts throughout the race and did not push hard, as my cardiologist recommended. The race went well considering the recent procedure.

At my next rehab phone appointment, the nurse asked me about my exercise schedule and went completely silent when I told her about running a marathon. Thinking she had not heard me correctly, she asked again about the distance. I got an earful from her and my cardiologist, who heard the news the next day. I told the nurse that, in my defense, I had cleared the run with my cardiologist; however, I admitted we never qualified the definition of a run in terms of mileage. She told me to stay at 10 kilometers max for a few months before attempting any longer races and until I got the clearance from my cardiologist.

Before Christmas, a few days after the marathon, I lifted a heavy box and aggravated an old injury of a herniated disk. This grounded me; I guess it was my body's way of telling me it needed some time to recover. The well-deserved break lasted three months before I could run again. With regular brisk walks, yoga and Tai-Chi, I recovered from my herniated disk and went back to training. Marathons and 50Ks followed and I delighted at being back on my running schedule. My cardiologist did not allow me to go beyond 50K for at least a year after my procedure and I had to stay at 70% performance. Moving to a new age division recently has helped me to place in most of my races.

One might ask why I persist with running even with all of the physical problems I have encountered, especially with my heart. Something magical occurs in the silence of nature; ultra-runner friends call it "nature bathing." In some races, the heat and the hills make it much easier to let go whatever is on my mind and force me to be present on the trails. From my Tai-Chi practice, I have learned to keep focused on the moment. I become alert to every sound and movement on the trails and running turns into meditation in motion. The endorphin rush makes the colors more vivid and nature becomes one continuous painting with hues hard to imitate by any master painter. Connecting to the energy of the earth brings about peace and harmony, which washes away all the fears of being on my own in the wilderness without seeing or talking to anyone for miles. There is power in that silence; a power that calls me to get back on the trail as soon as a race is over.

It has been said that running does not add years to your life, but it adds life to your years. When not running, I did not have any symptoms. My breathing came naturally and there was no sign of any heart issues. I had not been aware I had 95% blockage in my right artery. I only knew that, when running, I had difficulty breathing and my chest would get tight. I have a family history of heart disease and have taken cholesterol medicine for decades. I have treated my body like a race car, having regular annual check-ups and follow-ups whenever I felt any signs of trouble. I have learned to listen to my body through the years. This particular heart problem eluded any solution, but I stayed persistent in finding the reason for my shortness of breath, chest tightness and irregular heartbeat. At times, I strayed from the truth, wanting to believe alternative solutions. As a runner, I had blamed my breathing difficulties on the lack of conditioning. Ironically, although running could have killed me, it ended up saving my life. One other change has been made: To this day, my wife sighs in relief when I send her a text after every race that reads "Done."

EKG – An electrocardiogram (ECG or EKG) records the electrical signal from your heart to check for different heart conditions. Electrodes are placed on your chest to record your heart's electrical signals, which cause your heart to beat
https://www.mayoclinic.org/tests-procedures/ekg/about/pac-20384983#:~:text=An%20elec-trocardiogram%20(ECG%20or%20EKG,cause%20your%20heart%20to%20beat

Stress Test – A stress test, also called an exercise stress test, shows how your heart works during physical activity. Because exercise makes your heart pump harder and faster, an exercise stress test can reveal problems with blood flow within your heart.
https://www.mayoclinic.org/tests-procedures/stress-test/about/pac-20385234#:~:text=A%20stress%20test%2C%20also%20called,blood%20flow%20within%20your%20heart

CT Scan - A computerized tomography (CT) scan combines a series of X-ray images taken from different angles around your body and uses computer processing to create cross-sectional images (slices) of the bones, blood vessels and soft tissues inside your body. CT scan images provide more-detailed information than plain X-rays do
https://www.mayoclinic.org/tests-procedures/ct-scan/about/pac-20393675#:~:text=A%20computerized%20tomography%20(CT)%20scan,than%20plain%20X%2Drays%20do

Oxygen deprivation – asphyxia (ăs-fĭk'sē-ə) A condition in which an extreme decrease in the concentration of oxygen in the body accompanied by an increase in the concentration of carbon dioxide leads to loss of consciousness or death.
https://medical-dictionary.thefreedictionary.com/Oxygen+deprivation#:~:text=(%C4%83s%2Df%C4%ADk%E2%80%B2s%C4%93%2D,loss%20of%20consciousness%20or%20death

H.Pylori Bacteria Infection – *Helicobacter pylori* (*H. pylori*) is a type of bacteria. These germs can enter your body and live in your digestive tract. After many years, they can cause sores, called ulcers, in the lining of your stomach or the upper part of your small intestine. For some people, an infection can lead to stomach cancer.
https://www.webmd.com/digestive-disorders/urea-breath-test

IV - Intravenous (IV): 1) Into a vein. Intravenous (IV) medications are a solutions administered directly into the venous circulation via a syringe or intravenous catheter (tube).
https://www.rxlist.com/intravenous_iv/definition.htm

Code blue - indicates a medical emergency such as cardiac or respiratory arrest. Code red indicates fire or smoke in the hospital. Code black typically means there is a bomb threat to the facility. Hospitals are the most common institutions that use color codes to designate emergencies
https://www.healthline.com/health/code-blue#:~:text=Code%20blue%20indicates%20a%20medical,color%20codes%20to%20designate%20emergencies.

CPR – Cardiopulmonary Resuscitation is an emergency lifesaving procedure performed when the heart stops beating. Immediate CPR can double or triple chances of survival after cardiac arrest.
https://cpr.heart.org/en/resources/what-is-cpr

AED - An AED, or automated external defibrillator, is used to help those experiencing sudden cardiac arrest. It's a sophisticated, yet easy-to-use, medical device that can analyze the heart's rhythm and, if necessary, deliver an electrical shock, or defibrillation, to help the heart re-establish an effective rhythm.
https://www.redcross.org/take-a-class/aed/using-an-aed/what-is-aed#:~:text=An%20AED%2C%20or%20automated%20external,re%2Destablish%20an%20effective%20rhythm

Coronary Calcium Test - Also known as a CAC *test*, it involves a type of rapid X-ray called a CT scan. It takes cross-sectional images of the vessels that supply blood to the *heart* muscle, to check for the buildup of calcified plaque, which is composed of fats, cholesterol, *calcium* and other substances in the blood.
https://www.heart.org/en/news/2018/11/13/coronary-calcium-test-could-help-clarify-heart-disease-risk-and-control-cholesterol

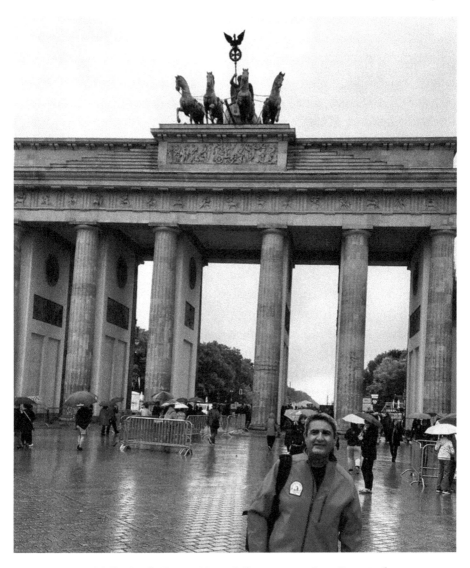

With Each Race New Adventures Are Created

One of my goals has been to run the Marathon Majors. The Majors currently consist of marathons in Boston, New York, Chicago, Sydney, Tokyo, London and Berlin. Now that I have completed Berlin, London is the last one left to finish my Majors goal. The Berlin Marathon 2019 had a total of 61,390 participants from 133 nations (and about 11,000 Breakfast-Run participants on the day before the marathon). 40,775 runners finished the race (28,443 men, 12,332 women). A new world record was missed by 2 seconds (with a time of 2:01:41).

On the morning of the marathon, a massive nervous energy could be felt at the starting line. Hours later, shivering runners straggled to the finish in the pouring rain. These moments represent some of my favorite parts of big road races, when I am most present to the energy of the crowd. At our dinner table the night before the race, someone offered a taste of a mystery fruit and I took the challenge (I should have known better). In one of the fastest courses in the world, my pace remained slow. The mystery fruit form the night before had upset my stomach. I felt uncomfortable, but I finished the race. I made the most of it by cheering the spectators and giving high-fives to the kids lining the course in the rain.

Although I stayed only four days, intuitively Berlin felt very familiar to me, as if I had lived there before. Having once been a divided city, Berlin had a distinct energy between what used to be East and West Berlin. Sometimes those differences arose just by crossing the street to the other side. A kind of darkness covered the city, even in the sunlight. I thought it might have to do with the past. The city had suffered through two World Wars, leaving a defeated nation with a resigned population that no longer craved wars. A piece of the wall separating East and West Berlin is kept for the tourists to visit. The bullet holes on a few monuments that I visited were kept intact. The tour guide mentioned the need for a remembrance of the past. As I touched the wall and ran my fingers through the broken pieces of bricks, I asked the tour guide if she referred to a past that remembered defeat or to one that reminded them not to prepare for another war. She did not have an answer. It seemed to me that, even though the Germany holds the most significant economic position in Europe, it feels inferior. Maybe the young can dream of victorious days ahead.

In 2015, a huge influx of refugees entered Europe to escape untenable situations in their own countries. For Berlin, this most recent challenge revolved around how these refugees would enculturate into German society. They came from the war-torn countries of Syria, Iraq and Afghanistan, whose cultures and belief systems were vastly different from those of Germany.

I knew of the recent international crisis that affected Berlin. This inspired me to seek out recent refugees for some interaction and I took the opportunity to engage with them beyond the marathon event. I made sure to take Uber for transportation so I would have an opportunity to meet and talk to them. Without exception, every Uber driver of mine turned out to be a recent refugee from the Middle East or Asia. I greeted them in Arabic and Farsi. The longing for their home, which they may never see again, resonated with me since I also immigrated to the United States from the Middle East over 40 years ago, and have been prevented from returning due to a change in power. Most greeted me warmly; they offered me sweets as is the custom in their culture, took the longest route to my destination and opened up to talk to me about their lives in this new home, their families, their pasts and their struggles. They had a lot to share. I actively listened to them but did not offer any thoughts or advice. They talked of how they have learned not to cross the invisible wall of marginalization in their new country. This may have to do with the zero tolerance of authorities for any type of conflict created by refugees. According to most of the drivers, the police actions have been swift, with a proven track record of deportations.

My observation of this small sample of drivers demonstrated the trauma of displacement, fear of authority, fear of losing their jobs as Uber drivers and hesitancy to fully assimilate. For now, they rely on their friends and insular communities and hope that their children will be the ones to break the barriers of marginalization. The children do not want to go back to their homeland. Because the families are tight knit, parents would always choose to stay with their children, although their longing for home creates a chronic anxiety which most of them may never acknowledge. A few of the children will grow to have a significant impact on the new land they know as home.

Running marathons around the world opens me up to a variety of experiences and interactions with people I normally would never know. In this case, the marathon became a vehicle for my being in Berlin during this time in history, when a massive migration had uprooted many people from war-torn countries and brought them to Germany.

As one of the drivers framed it, unless we learn how to take care of each other as human beings, we can all become refugees. In reflecting back on my Uber conversations, I consider that part of my trip to be almost more important than running another marathon.

Marathon Number 237
Berlin Marathon
September 2019

Enculturation - is the process by which people learn the requirements of their surrounding culture and acquire values and behaviors appropriate or necessary in that culture. ... Enculturation is related to socialization. In some academic fields, socialization refers to the deliberate shaping of the individual.
https://www.definitions.net/definition/Enculturation

Farsi - Is used as the local defining name for the Persian language, is the Arabized form of the word Parsi; the language sees widespread use in Iran, Afghanistan, Tajikistan and other regions of the former Persian empires.
https://en.wikipedia.org/wiki/Parsis

Marginalization - A spatial metaphor for a process of social exclusion in which individuals or groups are relegated to the fringes of a society, being denied economic, political, and/or symbolic power and pushed towards being 'outsiders'.
https://www.oxfordreference.com/view/10.1093/oi/authority.20110803100133827#:~:text=(sociology),pushed%20towards%20being%20'outsiders'

Active listening - is a technique that is used in counseling, training, and solving disputes or conflicts. It requires the listener to fully concentrate, understand, respond and then remember what is being said.
https://en.wikipedia.org/wiki/Active_listening

Refugee - One that flees, especially a person who flees to a foreign country or power to escape danger or persecution
https://www.merriam-webster.com/dictionary/refugee

Immigrant - A person who comes to a country to take up permanent residence
https://www.merriam-webster.com/dictionary/immigrant

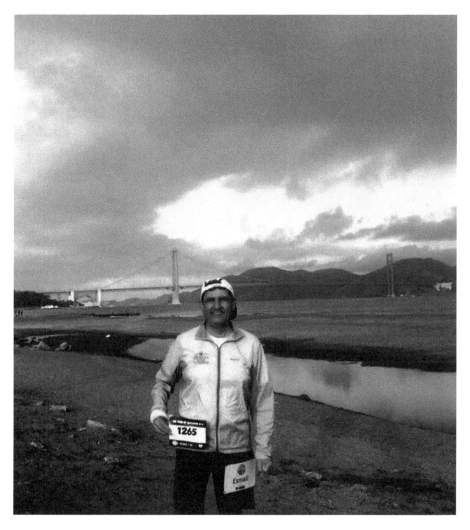

No Start, No Finish

1.06-mile loop, a random point selected close to the parking lot to lay the timing mat, an aid station set up by smiling volunteers, an old gentleman with a colorful turban cutting oranges and watermelon. Someone remarks that oranges never tasted so good. Each individual chooses to be out here for six, twelve or twenty-four hours, repeating the same course. Much like sitting in Meditation, practicing Yoga, chanting Buddhist Mantras, reciting Catholic prayers in weddings and funerals, or reading the sacred books of Jewish, Muslim, Christian and Hindu faiths. Does running make one spiritual or is spirituality manifested in running?

A brief conversation in the dark with a runner named Isaac who smiles as he asks for my name. After a short pause, he comments that we are all being watched over. An old friend and I drag our feet and, during one loop, she tells me about her life in the last seven years. She admits that she was ready to go home after a few loops, but it took her about fifteen miles to let go. "Some do not let go after fifteen years," I say to her. Maybe it is about being present, alone out there and alone together as we repeat the same loop in life, so that we can get it right. The distance is our choosing.

New Year's One Day
Crissy Field, San Francisco
December 31, 2014- January 1, 2015

CPSIA information can be obtained
at www.ICGtesting.com
Printed in the USA
JSHW012129170621
16011JS00003B/10